Praise for Fast to Faith: A 40-Day Awakening Program

"Dr. Tabatha Barber and her program are a gift from God, as is fasting—the Christian Bible says *"when* you fast", not *"if* you fast"—implying fasting is expected. God has also given us all of the foods we need to nourish our bodies. In her book, *Fast to Faith*, Dr. Tabatha takes you gently by the hand and walks you through her 40 day program. As you transition through the four phases of her program—Sunrise, Transition, Freedom, and Enlightenment—you'll reconnect with yourself—body, mind and spirit—while also growing deeper into your faith."

— Gin Stephens, *New York Times* best selling author of *Fast Feast Repeat* and host of two podcasts: *Intermittent Fasting Stories* and *Fast Feast Repeat Intermittent Fasting for Life*

"As someone deeply immersed in the world of holistic health and wellness, I've seen countless transformations, but Dr. Tabatha's journey stands out exceptionally. Observing her metamorphosis and the fervor with which she birthed *Fast to Faith* has been nothing short of awe-inspiring. With an unmistakable commitment, she seeks to empower women to embrace their most genuine selves and reach unparalleled health heights. Dive into this book and discover not just the undeniable benefits of whole foods and the power of fasting, but find a guide that nurtures your spirit and enriches your innermost being. *Fast to Faith* is more than a guide; it's a soulful journey."

— JJ Virgin, *New York Times* bestselling author, founder and CEO of *The Mindshare Collaborative*

"Whenever I have a difficult decision or time of struggle, I fast and pray. That is why I am so excited about this book, *Fast to Faith* by Dr. Tabatha Barber. In it she gives hope, inspiration and the path to the embodiment of true health– mind, body and spirit. Her own personal story is one every woman should hear. She truly is inspirational. One of the many reasons why I highly recommend this book is because Dr. Barber shares practical steps and relatable stories that help readers understand how they too can experience a transformation in their own spiritual and physical journey."

— Dr. Anna Cabeca, aka *The Girlfriend Doctor*, menopause expert and best-selling author of *The Hormone Fix*

"Dr. Tabatha's journey is nothing less than remarkable; her inspiring story embodies the loving, caring, compassionate physician that she is and the impact of her faith throughout her lifetime. The concept of fasting is not new or novel, it is a component of all the major religions and I love that Tabatha incorporates the transformative aspects of fasting, mind-body-spirit, into her new book. *Fast to Faith: A 40-Day Awakening* provides mental clarity and greater connection to your faith and your health."

— Cynthia Thurlow, NP, intermittent fasting and metabolic health expert, best-selling author of *The Intermittent Fasting Transformation* and host of *Everyday Wellness podcast*

"Dr. Tabatha understands the physical, mental, emotional and spiritual struggles we women face in this modern world. She explains complex medical concepts in a way that makes complete sense and reminds us that God created our bodies for health and vitality. When we connect to our body and soul, we connect to God. *Fast to Faith* is a simple, easy to digest program that harnesses the power of fasting to heal us and meditating on the word of God to find our strength to transform."

— Achina Stein DO, FACN, IFMCP, functional psychiatrist and author of *What If It's Not Depression?: Your Guide to Finding Answers and Solutions*

"*Fast to Faith* is a game-changing guide that empowers women to unlock their inner strength and faith. Dr. Tabatha Barber's *40-day Awakening* offers a powerful journey to reclaiming health, self-love, and a deeper discovery of faith and spirituality. With tangible insights and unwavering encouragement, this book is a must read for any woman looking to transform their life and embrace a newfound sense of purpose."

— Craig Siegel, founder of *CLS* coaching program, best-selling author of *The Reinvention Formula*, global speaker, and marathoner

"*Fast to Faith* is a truly transformative book that not only guides women in deepening their faith, but also equips them with the tools to conquer challenging obstacles. Dr. Tabatha's *40-Day Awakening* is a beacon of hope, helping women overcome stubborn food cravings, negative self-talk, and body shaming. Through her powerful insights, this book offers a roadmap to renewed health, self-acceptance, and a strengthened connection with God. It's a remarkable journey that every woman seeking a positive change in their life should embark upon."

— Tricia Nelson, emotional eating expert with over 1 million TEDx views and founder of healyourhunger.com

"*Fast to Faith: A 40-Day Awakening* is a divinely inspired journey that empowers women to regain control of their health, bodies, and faith. Through the transformative power of fasting, Dr. Barber guides women to conquer cravings, silence self-doubt, and break free from body shaming. Her personal journey, as a patient and a physician, shines through in her compassionate and transformative approach to healthcare. *Fast to Faith* is a must-read, and I'm confident it will make a profound impact on your life."

— Dr. Deb Matthew, best-selling author of *This Is Not Normal* and *Why Can't I Keep Up Anymore?*, international speaker, and owner of *Signature Wellness*

"*Fast To Faith* is a must-read for those seeking not just physical healing and personal growth, but a truly holistic transformation of mind, body, and spirit. Dr. Tabatha Barber is a distinguished medical doctor who shares her personal, inspirational journey of how faith led her into medicine and has been the guiding light through her own healing journey. Her commitment to sharing her wisdom is a testament to her passion for helping others lead healthier, happier, faith based lives. Dive into this book and embark on your own transformative journey with the guidance of a trusted expert in both medicine and faith."

— Jackie Bowker, CEO of *The Global Feel Better Institute*, international speaker, nutrition scientist, gut expert, and creator of the *Gut, Brain, Body Reset*

Fast to Faith

A 40-Day Awakening

Fast to Faith

A 40-Day Awakening

**Reconnect Your Body, Mind and Soul for Lasting
Weight Loss, Sustained Energy, and Unstoppable Strength**

Tabatha Barber, DO, FACOOG, NCMP, IFMCP

Published by Best Seller Publishing®, St. Augustine, FL
Best Seller Publishing® is a registered trademark.
Printed in the United States of America.
ISBN:978-1-962595-54-4

All scripture has been taken from the Holy Bible New International Version (NIV)

For more information, please write:
Best Seller Publishing®
1775 US-1 #1070
St. Augustine, FL 32084
or call 1 (626) 765-9750
Visit us online at: www.BestSellerPublishing.org

Disclaimer: Fasting can have potential risks and may not be suitable for everyone, especially those with certain medical conditions. Even though I am a physician, I am not your physician. Consulting with your own healthcare professional before attempting any fasting regimen is crucial to ensure safety and effectiveness.

Moment of Gratitude

I am so grateful for this journey called life, for the adversities, the joyous moments, and everything in between. I believe God has put a calling on my life and I have chosen to be obedient, no matter how uncomfortable or scary it may seem. I believe He is calling on you, too, and that is why you are reading this, so lean in, be curious, and FAITH IT!™

I want to publicly thank my family and friends for always loving me and reminding me to shine my light when I struggle and lose my perspective. I want to thank the thousands of women (and a few good men) who have entrusted me to be their physician during some of the hardest times and some of the most miraculous times. Lastly, I want to thank you for opening this book. Please know, I will always advocate for you (and all women) to have a voice and another choice when it comes to your body and your health!

Contents

Introduction: Why Me? 1

Part 1: Why Fasting Is Your Superpower From God

1 Clarify How Fasting Heals 17
2 Reconnect the Body, Mind, & Soul 29
3 Find Your Lost Intuition 41
4 Truth Behind Cravings 51
5 Change Your Physiology 71
6 Your Innate Intelligence 85
7 Frankenfoods Versus Faith Foods 97
8 Future Gazing with God 107
9 Prepare for Success 115
10 Honor God In All Aspects 125

Part 2: Start Your 40-Day Awakening

11 Begin with Sunrise - Days 1-10 141
12 Move into Transition Phase 2 - Days 11-20 161

13 Kickstart Your Freedom in Phase 3 – Days 21-30 181

14 Become Enlightened - Days 31-40 199

Part 3: Faithful Future

15 Thrive in Faith for Years to Come 215

Resources 223

Introduction: Why Me?

My mom used to say I was a wild child. It was Friday night parties, six hours of Saturday school detention, then church on Sundays.

When I was 16, I got pregnant and dropped out of high school. I had to go on food stamps and Medicaid, and I was assigned to a grumpy old doctor on the verge of retirement.

I remember having endless pelvis exams, getting shots, taking pills, and having procedures. Not one doctor or nurse asked for my permission, gave me options, or explained why they were doing what they were doing. I didn't have a voice or a choice when it came to my body.

I made it 42 weeks without any signs of labor, so I had to be induced. It dredged on for what felt like eternity. When my water broke, it was as green as pea soup.

"Is it supposed to be that color?" I asked timidly.

Up until then I hadn't questioned anything because they were wearing the white coats so I thought they knew best. But now, it wasn't just about me, it was about my unborn baby, and seeing pea-soup green scared me.

"Don't worry about it, see (pointing to the monitor), your baby is fine," the nurse said.

Trying to understand, I asked, "What do these squiggles printed on the paper mean?"

She snapped back, "That your baby is fine. Do you think we would just sit here if it wasn't?"

I mustered up the words, "I guess not."

After three and a half hours of trying to push my baby out, crying, and begging for a c-section because the pain was so excruciating, the doctor finally came in.

Finally, someone is going to help me. Thank you, God! I screamed in my head.

I'd been suffering alone. My boyfriend was asleep in the next room, and my mom had left to take care of her own kids. It was just me and my baby inside me who made it clear she didn't want to come into this scary world.

The doctor came in, draped my legs wide open over cold metal leg holders and prepped me. Suddenly, the relentless pain turned into a burning, searing, unbearable pain.

Clang! Clang!

As that sound of metal hit the floor it felt like knives piercing up and down my spine.

He had used forceps to deliver my daughter and tore me from front to back. I was never the same. I spent the next hour biting a wet washcloth, tears rolling down my face, while the doctor put me back together with shots and sutures. I focused instead on my crying daughter. What a soothing, beautiful sound.

I thought, Oh, I wish they would let me hold you, my sweet baby Ellie. I vow to never let you go through this alone or without options. I will do whatever it takes to give you a voice, a choice, support, and love.

God spoke to me that day. I heard Him clearly say, "You need to get your life together for you and your daughter. You need to use your voice to ask for the respect you deserve."

As it turned out, that doctor couldn't perform c-sections because he was a family practice doctor, not an obstetrician. That meant I had no choice of using another doctor or another method of delivery. I came out of that experience not only a mother, but also a woman—a woman on a mission.

I realized my daughter needed me to take charge of my life. I realized that women needed better options. I realized that I needed to learn how to use my voice and ask for the respect I deserved as a human being. And most importantly, I realized that I wasn't alone; the Holy Spirit was holding me the entire time, giving me strength, and showing me my purpose. God shows up in the darkness and shines His light upon us. He takes what was meant for our harm and turns it into good.

I could have felt sorry for myself and let that chapter limit my life, but I chose to listen to my higher power. Over the next many months, He kept whispering to me, "Take care of your body, it is a gift to be cherished. Find your voice. Help other women find their voice. Help other women keep their bodies safe. Figure out how to help women feel heard, safe, and supported."

Back to school

I relied on my faith and determination to find the courage to go back and get my GED (graduate equivalent diploma) and go to a community college with plans to become a nurse. I quickly learned how to study and realized I was capable of way more than I ever believed. I went from getting Cs and Ds in high school before I had Ellie, to getting straight As for two years.

One day I found myself telling my professor that I was dreaming of becoming a doctor.

"I think nurses are amazing and the work they do is so important, but I don't want to carry out someone else's orders, I want to make those decisions for myself. I wish I could be a doctor instead."

"You can," that professor said with complete confidence and in all seriousness.

Those two words changed my life.

"You believe I could do that?" I asked in shock.

"Without a doubt. And God put you on this path to do great things, to help women, so I know you will succeed. You could go to Michigan State like I did. I could write you a letter of recommendation," he offered.

That day when I heard my professor's belief in me and his reminder of what God was trying to do with my life, I found complete clarity. I know now that God was speaking to me through my professor. He uses the people in our life to do His work. No doubt He has used you at some point to influence another person's destiny.

After two years, I transferred to Michigan State University with two scholarships and did another four years of undergrad, majoring in physiology—the study of how the human body functions down to the cellular level and in response to the environment it's exposed to. I graduated with a bachelor's degree and high honors.

I only applied to one medical school because I didn't want to move my kindergartener, and I knew I wanted to go to an osteopathic medical school because they seemed to stress the importance of the mind-body connection. I got accepted into that medical school and became the physician that I had needed a decade prior. I became the doctor my daughter and other women needed—one who would talk to her patients, let them know the options available, and that they are not alone in their journey.

Please understand that I had no idea how I was going to do any of it. That's what it means to rely on God and on your faith.

Like Martin Luther King, Jr. said, "We don't have to see the whole staircase, just the first step."

> Have you had a moment that changed the trajectory of your future? Were you up for the challenge of stepping into your greatness? No worries, if you weren't. I promise another challenge will present itself and God will give you the opportunity, once again, to grow into the person you are meant to become. I believe you get as many chances as you need to step into your greatness and shine the way you were born to shine. My Fast to Faith: A 40-Day Awakening program is just that!

Living the life?

Fast forward 20 years. I am living the life of an attending physician; the life I worked so hard to create. The life I thought God wanted for me. I would wake up at 6am, rush around the house waking up my two babies, feeding them, packing their bags for daycare, taking a quick shower, and doing everything in my power to get to the office by 7:30am. No matter how hard I tried, I usually rolled in around 7:45 or 8am. By the time I got my computer up and running, answered some questions for my nurse, talked about the day's plan with my manager, and started seeing patients, I was already a half hour behind and I hadn't even "started my day."

For the next eight hours, I would rush through patient after patient trying to catch up, only to end up further and further behind. After all, I wanted to listen to my patients and actually try to help them, not just crank them through like an assembly line (which is what administration wanted me to do).

I almost never had time to eat lunch, and I often had to run to deliver a baby during my work day, only to make patients frustrated that they had to wait even longer. Many nights I had to scramble and find someone to pick up my kids from daycare because they were closing and I wasn't finished working. I barely had enough stamina to make it through the evening entertaining and caring for two rambunctious toddlers. Many nights, I had a babysitter sleep at my house because I was on call a lot and had to leave during the night for deliveries.

I was beyond sleep deprived. I was addicted to sugar and caffeine to stay awake and function every day. As you can imagine, this was not a sustainable way to live, nor was it rewarding.

I got to a point where I began having constant back pain and fatigue. I struggled while delivering babies. I could no longer sit on the edge of the bed with the laboring patient and help her push because it was too painful. I was also in pain the entire time I stood at the operating room table. When I finished a c-section or a hysterectomy, I wouldn't even be able to walk away from the table. I had to bend forward and spend two or three minutes trying to get my body to move and not be in excruciating pain. The hypocrisy was real. Here I was, the healthcare expert for women, and I was as unhealthy as it gets.

My body finally reached its breaking point and I went to the doctor. I was suffering from a herniated, ruptured disc in my lower back. My entire body was inflamed and angry. I saw the orthopedic surgeon and he told me that this had been going on for so long that I required surgery.

"How in the world am I going to not work for six weeks? Who's going to take care of my patients? Who's going to take care of my kids?"

It seemed impossible. I finally admitted defeat and accepted my fate. I had surgery and took six weeks off to heal. As soon as I went back to work, I was on call for five nights straight (to make up for being gone), and on night three, during a stressful delivery, I reinjured my back. I couldn't move, and I was devastated.

I just went through all of that for nothing. I'm right back where I started! What now? I thought.

I went back to the surgeon and he said, "Yep, you re-herniated. Now we need to put hardware in your back—rods and screws."

And then he jokingly added, "Back surgery is like Lay's potato chips, you can't have just one."

I thought, Dear God, I can't do this again. Please help me.

"Use your voice!" I heard God scream as if trying to wake me from a dream.

Dear God, help me!

And just like that, I woke up. My daughter's delivery from 25 years earlier flashed before me and I remembered how I vowed to God to protect the body he gave me.

"TIME OUT! More surgery? There has to be another choice," I demanded in a way that surprised both of us.

"Nope, not really," the surgeon said flippantly. "Unless you just want to live with the pain."

I didn't want to live in pain, but I didn't want to settle for his opinion, so I did the unthinkable. I finally listened to my intuition, used my voice, demanded there be another choice, and put myself first. I stopped obsessively worrying about my patients, my colleagues, or even my family. I heard God clearly say to me, "Figure this out. You have gone astray. You are not living into the purpose I have set out for you. You have important things to do and more band-aid surgeries are not the answer. I have already given you the tools to heal your body and be well. Trust me."

It felt right to be in alignment with God again. He is truly the only one who has had my body, my rights, and my wishes in mind.

I didn't schedule surgery. I left confused, but determined to find a different way. I realized conventional medicine was failing me, so I started researching outside of my normal journals and sources and was amazed to find an entire world of wellness and prevention out there that I knew nothing about.

I stumbled upon Dr. Amy Myers and watched a video she made about autoimmune thyroid. I thought, *Hey wait, I have that. Why is that an issue?*

As I listened, she reminded me of how physiologic processes in the body create health or disease. She went on to explain inflammation and how having an autoimmune disease is essentially having an overactive immune system that is attacking your own body. But then she went deeper.

She talked about how our gut is the root cause of this autoimmune condition and how it causes so many symptoms—fatigue, eczema, brain fog, weight gain, joint pain, constipation, and diarrhea. She was listing everything I was feeling. She talked about how she not only went to medical school, but also went on to study functional medicine and that was how she became an expert in gut health and autoimmune thyroid disease.

I had never heard of functional medicine, but I knew my next mission! I found the Cleveland Clinic's Institute for Functional Medicine and started consuming everything I could get my hands on. I read *Eat Fat, Get Thin* by Dr. Mark Hyman, did exactly what he recommended, and started feeling better. I listened to him in every way I could—on podcasts, webinars, masterclasses, and docuseries.

I found hope. I found answers. Most importantly, I was reminded that I was a child of God and that through Him all things were possible. I had forgotten that powerful fact. The way I was living was not nurturing my soul, it was slowly killing it a little bit every day.

Nothing left to give

> Jesus looked at them and said, "With man this is impossible, but with God all things are possible." –Matthew 19:26

I enrolled in the Cleveland Clinic's Institute for Functional Medicine (IFM) courses and began studying. Everything I learned, I applied to myself. I was my own guinea pig and it was working. My brain started thriving again—I was able to remember things, I had energy to get through the day, and I didn't need a nap anymore. I lost 20 pounds in three months, and my back pain was lessening.

The other huge piece of the process was that I took four months off work and focused on my health like it was my full-time job. By the end of the four months, I was a changed person. My body had regained healthy function, my mind gained clarity, my soul found hope, and how I approached my patients' problems was forever changed.

I realized the way I was living—go, go, go, and putting everyone else first—had depleted my body so severely that it was struggling to function. I had nothing left to give.

I realized the way I was practicing medicine–everything I was doing to my patients, like covering up their symptoms with pills and surgery–was actually causing their bodies to have more issues. I was no better than the old doctor who delivered my daughter, who didn't listen or give me a choice.

I had to face the hard truth: Our medical system is broken. It breaks well-meaning doctors who enter it, and it breaks patients and keeps them broken, so they are stuck there, never to see their health or vitality again. The medical system has trained us to believe that our bodies are just separate compartments that don't interact or affect one another, and worse, that our mind and soul don't influence our body's physical state. We are also trained to believe that the body will inevitably have disease and decay and we just need to accept that fate.

Nothing could not be further from the truth!

As a physician, I was trained to look for disease. If there is no diagnosable disease that insurance would cover, then you get rid of the symptom that the patient is complaining about. But I could no longer view my patients' complaints as an annoyance to cover up or get rid of. In fact, those complaints were messages, warning signs from the body that something was going on that wasn't being addressed.

Physiologically, the body gives you signs when there is dysfunction somewhere that needs to be corrected. I finally understood and believed what I was told on the first day of medical school: The founding father of osteopathic medicine, Dr. Andrew Taylor Still, said that the body has the innate ability to heal and the physician just needs to guide that process.

Why had I forgotten that?

Doctors of osteopathic medicine (DO) were merged with medical doctors (MD) in the 1980s, which meant that the holistic, integrative training that set DOs apart from MDs was eventually blurred and left behind. DOs melted into the world of conventional medicine and focused their training on disease, just like the MDs. After my first year of medical school, I was in the same boat as the MD students. There was no more talk about innate intelligence, homeostasis, mind-body connection, or wellness.

Studying functional medicine was like going back to medical school, but learning about the body the way it should be

taught—by focusing on how the body functions, how it interacts with the world around it, how the bacteria, viruses, yeast,
parasites, and environmental pollutants affect us, how the body
reacts to stressors both physical and mental, and how all of our
systems are so intricately interconnected.

Our systems are not working in silos like conventional medicine would have you believe with all their -ologists (i.e., the cardiologists, gastroenterologists, dermatologists, gynecologists).
Everything about how our conventional medical system is struc-
tured is designed to keep us sick and focused on disease. I did
not accept that fate, and I don't want you to either. We need
to focus on true return of function (healing), wellness, and
prevention. That requires asking why. When a patient tells me
her complaints, it's my job to ask, "Why is she feeling that? Why
are her periods heavy? Why is she having severe headaches?"
Not to just spend five minutes finding a drug that will suppress
her symptoms and most likely cause a new one.

Once I began practicing this way, I no longer fit into the
conventional "care" model. I wasn't allowed to spend more time
with patients to actually ask the questions I needed to put all the
pieces together. I wanted to ask about what they were putting
into their body every day, how they were sleeping, what type of
stress they were dealing with, whether or not they were exercising
or moving their body, or if they were taking time to nurture their
relationships with others and with themselves.

The answers to those types of questions hold the key to
true healing. We can't ever fix conditions like endometriosis if
we are focused on trying another pill or having another surgery,
because we are not supporting the body back to homeostasis.
The disorder and dysfunction continue, multiply, and spill over
into other systems because every system impacts the other.

Why is that? Because the endocrine system oversees all
our systems. The endocrine system refers to the collection

of glands that produce, secrete, and manage hormones. This includes your glands in your brain (the hypothalamus, pituitary, pineal), adrenal glands, pancreas, thyroid, thymus, and ovaries. So, this system and these glands affect your brain and nervous system, your digestive system, your metabolism, your reproductive system, your cardiovascular system, etc.

When I was living my stressed-out, sleep-deprived, nutrient-deplete, mindless life, my adrenal glands were keeping me alive by producing excessive amounts of cortisol and adrenaline. Those are our two main stress response hormones. I was taxing my pancreas, requiring excess insulin production to manage all the sugar and processed foods I was mindlessly consuming. My immune system was attacking my own thyroid and preventing it from functioning properly because I had an autoimmune process going on, being fueled by all the gluten I was consuming, and my ovaries were responding by downregulating their function. We'll talk about this more in the coming chapters, so you can start to figure out what is going on in your own body.

No way to thrive in survival mode

Here's the deal, you can't be in survival mode and thrive mode at the same time. Our bodies were designed to be in homeostasis and procreate. God created us not only to survive, but also to thrive. Our souls–our true selves–are here in these bodies to have a human experience and how you tend to your body directly impacts the experience you have, the lessons you learn, the wisdom you gain, and your ability to love, nurture others, and make a greater impact on this world.

I truly believe that God wants us to leave this world better than we found it, so caring for your body first is essential for you to glorify the Lord and live into your purpose. We do that by reconnecting our physical body with what our mind is thinking and what our soul is craving.

Let my life be the proof, the proof of your love. –From the song "The Proof of Your Love" by For King & Country

Part 1

Why Fasting Is Your Superpower From God

*"To eat when you are sick
is to feed your illness."*

–Hippocrates

Chapter 1

Clarify How Fasting Heals

Let's go back 20+ years to when I was a medical student in East Lansing, Michigan. There I was in my short white coat (the short coat denotes a lesser rank in the hierarchy, so once you graduate and become a full-fledged physician, you graduate to the long white coat) doing my externship in the hospital. Each month we rotated to a different specialty to get an idea of which area of medicine we liked and what might be good at. We rotated between internal medicine, the ER, the OB/GYNs, the pediatricians, the surgeons, the urologists, etc.

I had many experiences that caused me to question how God "fit" into our medical system. I was raised to believe He was the ultimate healer, but now I was in a world where I was being told that I was the healer and that all the doctors training me were the healers.

I remember my surgical rotation in particular. I would wake up at 4:30am every morning to make sure I was at the hospital seeing patients by 5am. I needed to see every patient on the census before the resident did and they needed to see the patient before the attending physician did, which was usually around 7am. It was a high stress situation because if you didn't see a patient, you got called out in front of everyone at the morning meeting and were verbally desecrated.

"You're worthless. How do you expect to become a doctor and heal people when you can't even get out of bed!" is what we would hear.

So, I made sure I saw the patients and stuck around when the residents saw them because they would teach me things. They taught me how to take care of a patient "postoperatively," meaning someone who had just had surgery. One important piece I learned was that a patient had to fast for at least 12 hours before surgery and then after surgery they weren't allowed to eat right away.

There were three reasons for this. Number one, the anesthesia medications often make patients nauseous and if they vomited, they could aspirate and develop pneumonia. The second reason is that a patient's gastrointestinal system slows down significantly from the anesthesia and surgical manipulation of the bowels, so food would not be easily digested during recovery. The third and most important reason for fasting before surgery was that a patient's body needed to conserve resources to focus on healing, and when we eat, it slows down our healing process. Most patients were not even hungry after surgery, they just wanted to rest. Usually by the second day they would start feeling hungry and ask if they could eat. This was a good sign that their body was recovering from surgery.

We (the residents and students) actually had to write fasting as an order for the nurses to follow. The patient wasn't allowed to even drink water until the doctor wrote an order to allow it. This made me think: *We are using fasting as a prescription to help the patient heal.*

Since then, I have written NPO orders thousands of times to aid in the patient's healing. NPO is doctor's shorthand for "nothing by mouth." It comes from the Latin "nil per os." Man has known since the beginning of time that fasting heals.

What happens during fasting

Fasting refers to the act of abstaining from food for a certain amount of time; this can range from hours to days. We all fast when we are sleeping and some of us purposefully fast for longer. When you are not eating, therefore, you are fasting. Many people regularly fast every day without realizing it. For example, if you don't eat until two hours after you wake up, then you have been fasting since you stopped eating the night before.

Fasting has become a popular trend and there are many variations of it. Some people are afraid of the idea of fasting because they envision Jesus fasting for 40 days and 40 nights, never eating once. That is an extreme case and not what I'm talking about. I want you to embrace the idea of fasting for a period of time, and I am going to teach you why it should be part of your daily life.

Intermittent fasting refers to purposefully selecting the times when you will fast and usually involves intermittent cycles of different lengths of time. There have been popular diets encouraging only eating one meal per day, or fasting two times per week, or eating during a certain time frame each day. The key is that you are choosing to avoid eating for a designated amount of time.

Time-restricted feeding (TRF) is the term used to describe the time when you are eating, called your eating window. A popular method called 16/8 refers to fasting for 16 hours, followed by only eating during an eight-hour window. This method works nicely in most people's daily lives.

This program uses a variation of multiple fasting methods. I brought together the best of all practices to give you maximum results with the fewest challenges; those that are often encountered with strict, single-focused plans.

Fasting has amazing healing properties. When we stop intaking food, our pancreas stops making insulin, our organs stop making enzymes and chemicals to break down the food, the stomach and intestines stop requiring energy for digestion, and our body gets a chance to focus on other activities like healing.

Did you catch that? Our digestive system requires energy in the form of adenosine triphosphate (ATP) to digest our food. Eating is a lot of work for your body and we are asking it to do that work way too often.

When we stop eating, we can focus on healing.

When we eat, we are in a "fed state." When we fast, we are in a "fasted state." This time of fasted-state allows our body to use that ATP or energy elsewhere to heal. I call this "cleaning house." This is when our body gets to work and starts repairing itself at the level of the cells. This is the process of autophagy.

Autophagy is a cellular process that plays a crucial role in maintaining cellular health and homeostasis. The term autophagy comes from the Greek words "auto" (self) and "phagy" (eating), meaning "self-eating." It's an innate process by which cells destroy and recycle damaged organelles, proteins, and other cellular components.

Autophagy serves several critical functions within the cell:

1. Maintains cellular integrity: Autophagy removes damaged or malfunctioning organelles and proteins, thereby maintaining cellular health and preventing the accumulation of harmful substances.

2. Recycles nutrients: When the cell undergoes stress, such as a nutrient deficiency or lack of energy (ATP), autophagy enables the recycling of cellular components to provide essential building blocks and energy for the cell to survive.

3. Immune response: Autophagy is involved in the elimination of pathogens inside the cell. It also presents foreign antigens to immune cells to help the body fight against infection.

4. Cell differentiation: Autophagy plays a role in how stem cells decide what to become during development.

5. Cell quality: By removing damaged or misfolded proteins, autophagy helps prevent the accumulation of broken DNA and organelles that can lead to various neurodegenerative diseases, like Parkinson's disease and multiple sclerosis (MS).

Autophagy usually occurs after 24-48 hours of fasting. During this time, our body starts to break down and get rid of old cells–cells with broken DNA snippets, cells that are trying to go rogue and grow abnormally. Those are the ones that eventually lead to tumors, both benign and cancerous. Those are also the cells that are inflamed and are unable to hear a hormone signal. We all have inflammation, but the degree to which our body can combat and reverse it is very individualized as is the amount that inflammation affects our body's ability to function.

Cell signaling

Have you been told that your labs are normal, but you don't feel normal?

Almost every patient I have seen tells me that she doesn't understand how her labs can be fine, "...because I don't feel fine."

Not feeling fine is becoming the new norm. Women tell me they feel run down, they struggle to think clearly, they don't sleep well, they are carrying extra weight, and they feel anxious and/or depressed and can't figure out why. It's a recurring theme for many women. So, what exactly is going on?

All the trillions of cells that make up our body have receptors on them. The receptors act like locks, that when activated or unlocked, cause processes to happen, like opening a door to be able to walk inside. The receptors are designed in such a way that only certain hormones actually fit into it, like how specific keys fit into specific locks. Not all keys will turn and unlock a door. But even if you have the right key, if the key is bent or the lock has been damaged and the key doesn't fit properly, you can't unlock the door.

The same thing happens in our body. Even if our body is able to make enough estrogen or thyroid hormone, for example, that doesn't mean our cells can hear the signal that those hormones want to send. If our cells are inflamed, it damages the receptor (like a damaged lock), and the hormones (the key) can't bind to the cell and send their signal.

CELL RECEPTOR AND HORMONE SIGNAL

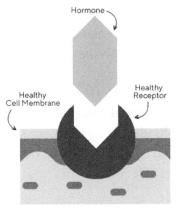

healthy HORMONE receptor cell

The hormone fits perfectly into the receptor to send the signal.

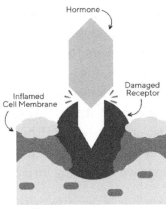

damaged HORMONE receptor cell

The hormone can't fit into the receptor to send the signal.

It's important to put our body into a fasted state on a regular basis to allow time for our body to clear out those damaged, poorly functioning cells and reverse the inflammation that was caused by our daily toxic living.

> *"Have mercy on me, O God, according to your unfailing love; according to your great compassion blot out my transgressions. Wash away all my iniquity and cleanse me from my sin." –Psalm 51:1-2*

Frankenfoods

Fasting, without a doubt, is the healthiest way to build your faith. I have encountered many people who claim to honor and love God, but do not show it in their actions toward their body. I was one of those people for a very long time.

God gives us one house for our earthly endeavor. We don't get to trade it in and get a new one if we abuse or destroy it. Because of that, He gave our bodies innate intelligence and incredible healing powers to survive the abuse He knew we would subject it to as humans.

It's time for us to honor God by honoring the body He gifted us.

We must stop treating it like a disposable garbage can. We must stop shoving in the Frankenfoods, giving in to our sugar, caffeine, and alcohol addictions, and truly think about how the things we're putting into our bodies affect us.

My definition of Frankenfoods is this: All the highly-processed foods in boxes and bags that didn't grow in the ground or have a mama. It's food that was created in a factory and has little to no nutritional value, yet we act like it's food, so we consume it 5-20 times a day to satisfy our taste buds and stop the hunger cravings. Think about the fact that we can eat an entire bag of chips, yet we can't eat more than a bowl of broccoli. The broccoli nourishes and satisfies us, the chips do not.

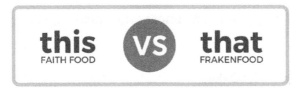

this FAITH FOOD	vs	that FRAKENFOOD
Wild Caught Fish & Sea Food		Fish Sticks
Grass-Fed Beef		Fast Food Hamburgers
Free Range Organic Chicken		Chicken Nuggets
Olive Oil & Vinegar		Cheap Salad Dressings
Whole Fruit		Canned Fruit Cocktail
Block of Real Aged Cheddar		Canned Cheese
Coffee & Tea		Starbucks Frappuccino

Examples of Frankenfoods: cereal, breakfast bars, oversized bagels, most bread, Pop Tarts, most yogurts, Starbucks coffee drinks, coffee creamers, margarine, donuts, Little Debbies, packaged baked goods, Slimfast products, most salad dressings, mac 'n' cheese, Velvetta, Hamburger Helper, frozen pizzas, pizza rolls, bagel bites, frozen dinners, fast food (like McDonalds, Burger King, Taco Bell, and Arby's), pop (soda), diet pop, sports drinks, Gatorade, energy drinks, Doritos, potato chips, pretzels, Oreos, cookies, candy, hot dogs, bologna, vegan meat and burgers, movie popcorn, Cheez Whiz, Cheez-its, crackers, ramen, fruit snacks, and the list goes on and on.

If you microwave these toxic foods in plastic, they become even more toxic—frozen meals, single mac 'n' cheese bowls, ramen in Styrofoam containers, and microwave popcorn are the worst.

Don't eat a SAD diet!

Frankenfoods are the basis of our Standard American Diet (SAD). The SAD diet refers to the highly processed foods that have little to no nutritional value, and are very high in carbohydrates, sugar, and inflammatory oils.

The majority of grains, corn, and soy in the U.S. are genetically modified and doused with pesticides and herbicides, which are known carcinogens (cancer causing agents).[1] This farming practice was first started to yield a higher amount of crop in a shorter period of time, but these foods have been so altered that our body no longer recognizes them. Our body sees these foods as foreign and because of this, our immune system goes on the attack when we eat them. Unfortunately, this has created an entire society of people with overactive, confused immune systems. This has led to the development of novel food allergies[2], an array of food sensitivities, staggering increases in autoimmune diseases[3], and other inflammatory diseases from chronic leaky gut, which I will explain later.

The SAD diet is driven by fast-food chains and highly processed foods that require minimal effort to prepare. They mass-produce their meat and dairy products with growth hormones and antibiotics to yield a higher quantity of food, which, in turn, destroys any nutrition that could be derived from

---

[1]   Mostafalou S, Abdollahi M. Pesticides: an update of human exposure and toxicity. Arch Toxicol. 2017 Feb;91(2):549-599. doi: 10.1007/s00204-016-1849-x. Epub 2016 Oct 8. PMID: 27722929
[2]   Origins of peanut allergyArchives of Disease in Childhood 2003;88:694.
[3]   Autoimmunity may be rising in the United States. U.S. Department of Health and Human Services & National Institute of Environmental Health Sciences (NIEHS). April 8, 2020 (Online Article)

those foods. These are known to affect our growth as humans, cause leaky gut, and disrupt our microbiomes.

The SAD diet also contains numerous unsafe chemicals that God never intended us to consume. We created them in a lab and it turns out that they are toxic to our body and contribute to the rise in chronic disease.

In March 2023, *Consumer Reports* wrote an article titled, "5 Dangerous Ingredients That Are In Our Food But Shouldn't Be" and in it they explain how they are co-sponsoring a bill with the Environmental Working Group (EWG) to ban certain food chemicals. The bill is now being debated in the California State Assembly, and if passed, would ban five chemicals from being used as additives in food and drinks sold in the state. This could have far-reaching effects for consumers throughout the country.

The substances—brominated vegetable oil, potassium bromate, propylparaben, Red Dye No. 3, and titanium dioxide—have each been linked to serious health problems, including a higher risk of cancer, nervous system damage, hyperactivity, and other behavioral problems. All have been banned by regulators for use in food in Europe.[4]

The SAD diet contains minimal vegetables and fruits, hence minimal fiber, antioxidants, or phytonutrients. I call these God foods and they are missing from our SAD diets. God created foods that not only nourish us, but also heal us, and we need to get back to eating those foods.

Our diet has strayed so far from what God planned for us that our bodies are rebelling. They are struggling to function because we contaminate and bombard them every single day with way too much sugar, way too many carbohydrates in the form of

---

4   "5 Dangerous Ingredients That Are in Our Food but Shouldn't Be: California has passed the Food Safety Act, the first law in the U.S. to ban harmful chemicals from foods," By Scott Medintz, March 20, 2023. Consumer Reports, Inc. (Online Blog)

highly processed GMO grains, and way too many toxins that we've created in the lab. There are more than 10,000 chemicals allowed by the FDA that are added into our food products[5], and many of these chemicals have been banned in other countries. We are the last country to admit that what we are consuming is killing us.

We have become a society of mindless consumers and many of us are so busy and overwhelmed with our busy day-to-day lives that we have lost the understanding of what it means to nourish our bodies. Many of us are living in a disconnected state; what our mind is thinking, what our soul is craving, and what our body is doing are often three different things. It's time to reconnect our trinity.

Have you felt dissatisfied and discouraged with your relationship with food? Have you felt frustrated with your body?

Keep reading!

---

[5]   AREAS OF FOCUS: TOXIC CHEMICALS: Food Chemicals. Environmental Working Group (Online Resource)

Chapter 2

Reconnect the Body, Mind, & Soul

Alex is a great example of the power that comes from reconnecting your body and mind with your soul. She is a 40-year-old woman who started working with me because she wanted to lose weight. Beyond her weight issues, she had spent her whole life struggling with depression and anxiety. Alex had been on Lexapro, a medication given for anxiety and depression, for over a decade with increasing and decreasing doses, trying to feel better. She explained to me that the medication made her feel numb inside, to the point where she didn't cry anymore. She explained that she was in therapy to learn boundaries and self-worth.

"My worth was wrapped up in my job and my ability to produce. It's caused a lot of stress for many years," she told me.

She was worried that all the stress had affected her health. She was at the point where she had no energy.

"I sleep for 10 or 12 hours and still need coffee to function," she had admitted to me.

We did a saliva testing to evaluate her 24-hour cortisol pattern. Her cortisol and DHEA production were so low that I diagnosed her with stage 3 adrenal dysfunction (previously called adrenal fatigue). I explained to her the connection between her thoughts and what she believes and how her body functions. She did my FTF online program and her transformation was incredible.

She said, "Since doing Fast to Faith, I believe in my body again. I know it's capable of so much more than I ever believed. I did a three-day water fast and I can now skip meals and not end up in the drive-through. That is huge. Understanding the difference between our psychological needs and our bodies' needs has been powerful."

Mind-Body connection

Everything you think, believe, and feel affects the physiology going on in your trillions of cells that make up your tissues, your organs, your systems—that make up your body.

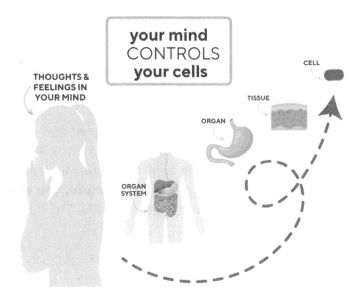

Your body operates according to the input it receives from your brain. Your brain is an organ that operates according to what your mind tells it to do. Your mind operates according to the input it receives from your soul and all the external stimuli from your environment (the universe). This input is either driven from dark energy and negativity (often referred to as the enemy) or from light energy and positivity, whom I call God.

Your brain is a computer and your mind is the computer program. It will do what you tell it. The brain continually tells the cells in your body to be congruent with your thoughts. If, for example, your thoughts are focused on negative things like being tired or in pain, it will produce chemicals and reactions to validate those thoughts and feelings. You will be kept in a vicious cycle of discomfort. If, on the other hand, you tell it to focus on positive things like joy, effortless movement, and healing, then it will tell your body to create those chemical messages.

This well-established psychological phenomenon known as "confirmation bias" explains how our brains have a bias towards seeking confirmation of our existing beliefs. This means we tend to favor information that confirms or supports our preexisting beliefs or values while ignoring or discounting information that contradicts those beliefs.[6,7]

It turns out we have way more authority over how our body feels and functions than the medical establishment will have you believe. God wants you to be in control and be mindful. I truly believe, **if you change what you tell your mind, you change what is possible for your health and your life.** The Bible tells us this in Romans 12:2:

> *Do not conform to the pattern of this world, but be transformed by the renewing of your mind. Then you will be able to test and approve what God's will is—His good, pleasing, and perfect will.*

When you have an on-going emotional relationship with God your cells hear those words and receive chemical messages from the feelings of hope and faith that you feel. Reading the Bible and nourishing your mind with the living, breathing Word has an incredible impact on your physical health.

According to research explained in the book *How God Changes Our Brain*, "Intense prayer and meditation permanently change numerous structures and functions in the brain—altering your values and the way you perceive reality." Their neuroscience research consisted of doing brain-imaging studies to examine

---

6   Wason, P. C. (1960). On the Failure to Eliminate Hypotheses in a Conceptual Task. Quarterly Journal of Experimental Psychology, 12(3), 129-140. DOI: 10.1080/17470216008416717

7   Nickerson, R. S. (1998). Confirmation bias: A ubiquitous phenomenon in many guises. Review of General Psychology, 2(2), 175–220. DOI: 10.1037/1089-2680.2.2.175

how various religious and spiritual practices, such as prayer, can influence the brain's activity and potentially lead to positive psychological and physiological changes. They explain the benefits of spiritual practices on mental health, stress reduction, and overall well-being.

As a child of God and a triple board-certified physician, I believe that He created our bodies with innate intelligence that is so sophisticated that we have only cracked the surface of how it works. What I do know for certain is that God created us to fast and to feast.

> "Even now," declares the LORD,
> "return to me with all your heart,
> with fasting and weeping and mourning." –Joel 2:12

Show your love for God and your body—FAST!

As already mentioned, fasting is the act of abstaining from food for a period of time. Fasting reminds us of our flesh, of our desires, and of our shortcomings as human beings. Fasting is meant to bring us closer to God. He wants us to rely on Him every day, in everything we do. That's what it means to have a relationship with Him.

I figured this out as I laid in my bed, unable to move for seven days after I reinjured my back. I told you how I went to the surgeon and was told I needed more surgery, but I didn't tell you how I was bedridden prior to that, unable to function.

As I lay there, surviving on muscle relaxers and pain killers, only being carried to the toilet by my husband a few times a day, I started to think about the fact that I had barely eaten anything in a week. Normally, I would turn to food during stressful times or lonely times. I ate when I was bored, when I was too stressed to think, or when I was lonely. I also ate when I was happy. Eating filled me emotionally on so many levels, or so I thought. It was a false satisfaction. This time, food couldn't fix the situation.

As I lay there, unintentionally fasting, I was in constant communication with God, crying out to Him to heal me, asking why He would let this happen to me. I felt betrayed. But something inside me told me to stop acting like a victim and search the Bible for words about healing. I was led to a scripture in the Old Testament that sparked a new idea.

> *There, by the Ahava Canal, I proclaimed a fast, so that we might humble ourselves before our God and ask him for a safe journey for us and our children, with all our possessions. I was ashamed to ask the king for soldiers and horsemen to protect us from enemies on the road, because we had told the king, "The gracious hand of our God is on everyone who looks to him, but his great anger is against all who forsake him." So we fasted and petitioned our God about this, and he answered our prayer.*
>
> *–Ezra 8:21-23*

Instead of focusing on the fact that I hadn't eaten in days or that I was in constant pain and unable to walk, I started focusing on how powerful God really could be if I just believed. I started asking Him to give me strength, show me how to overcome this situation, how to get healthy, and how to stop living in constant pain.

It was during those dark days that I came to this realization and deep understanding of how our body functions and how our soul and the Holy Trinity are connected to how it functions. I was innately fasting not only to heal my body, but also to turn my focus to God and look to Him for comfort, nourishment, healing, and the answers I so needed.

From then on, I became fascinated with fasting and how abstaining from food, not letting bodily sensations drive my decisions, and focusing on the positives instead of the negatives helped my mind to connect with feelings and energy outside of and beyond my physical body. It increased my ability to connect with the energy of the universe and the power of our creator. It was from these experiences that I learned the power of fasting.

I wrote my first book, *From White Trash to White Coat*, and most of this book you're reading in a fasted state because I gain so much mental clarity from abstaining from food. I have a more direct channel to allow the Holy Spirit to speak to me and work through me when my physical body isn't distracted by eating and digesting food.

Being in a fasted state means that I stop eating around 7pm and then I don't eat again until I break my fast the next day. Some days that is at 10am or even as late as 4pm depending on the situation.

I'm going to teach you the benefits of shorter fasts, called time-restricted feeding (TRF) and longer fasts.

Along with fasting, I also talk to God throughout my whole day, every day, thanking Him for little things, asking for guidance on the path that I know He has set out for me, and asking Him for strength to get through things that I alone cannot get through on my own.

Fasting is a great way to show God that you need Him and it's a great way to get your health back on track.

Body-Soul connection

> "Fasting is one of the greatest aspects of your prayer. When fasting is not added to your prayer, it is robbed of its potential power." -Benjamin Suulola

Learning how to fast didn't come easy for me, but fortunately I was learning functional medicine during this time. This concept of root cause medicine taught me that my terrible diet had me on a sugar roller coaster day and night. Once I learned the tools to get off the sugar roller coaster and stay off, I found freedom and health!

Throughout my healing journey, fasting has been the ultimate tool to hit the reset button and move the needle when it comes to my chronic conditions. I now teach my patients to use the healing properties of fasting through their journeys and have created this transformational program that gives you back the power over your body, your mind, and your soul's future.

While I was incorporating fasting and functional medicine into my healing journey, I was also studying the living, breathing Word of the Bible and quantum physics. What I figured out was that when you fast your body and nourish your mind according to the Word of God, you feed your soul and move toward health and healing.

Why is fasting more important than ever?

- According to the CDC, over the past 20 years (from 2000 to 2020), the number of obese people in the U.S. increased from 30.5% to 41.9%. That is close to half the population! Which side are you on?

- Obesity often correlates to conditions like heart disease, stroke, type 2 diabetes, and certain types of cancer. These are among the leading causes of *preventable*, premature death.

- The estimated annual medical cost of obesity in the U.S. was nearly $173 billion in 2019.

Thanks to these startling statistics, I started incorporating TRF, which is the most common form of fasting, into my patients' prescription plans. This consisted of patients eating only within an 8-10-hour window most days. I then taught them to do carb-cycling, which is a great way to stimulate your metabolism and break through weight loss plateaus (more to come on that later). Then, I started an online group program for women, teaching them how to fast and how to go from being a "sugar burner" to becoming a "fat burner."

I will explain the importance of this in Chapter 3, but please don't skip ahead because I am going to explain some foundational information that is crucial to your understanding of what is happening and why so many of us struggle with weight loss resistance and weight regain. I want you to be done with yo-yo dieting.

Eventually–and this is the most important part and what prompted me to write this book–I taught the women in my group not only the health benefits of fasting, but also the spiritual benefits they needed. We all need to nourish and heal our soul— that is what it means to be human.

I started asking women to do the emotional and spiritual work that I had done to heal myself. Their results went from great to outstanding. They not only lost weight, had more energy and brain clarity, and slept better, but they also liked themselves again, felt motivated and confident to pursue dreams they had been ignoring, felt comfortable in their own skin, and felt connected to God again, and for some women, for the first real time. This spilled over into every aspect of their lives. Their relationships became stronger, they broke through plateaus in their professional lives, and found joy in the simple things again.

I got to see first-hand over and over that true healing and transformation doesn't come from making physical changes alone. It comes from the Holy Trinity. It comes from listening to your intuition (the Holy Spirit), learning radical self-acceptance by modeling Christ's unconditional love and forgiveness *toward yourself*, and nurturing an on-going relationship with God. This distinct difference is the reason I am writing this book.

The mission God laid out for me was not just to deliver babies and do hysterectomies, it was also to create change. It was to give women control of their health and their bodies. God said to me, "Teach women the power of faith. Teach them to not only heal their bodies, but also to heal their souls. Teach them how to become whole."

The easiest way to take back control of your body and your health is to fast in a way that awakens your soul and strengthens your faith. I'm going to teach you this. You will learn to fast for physical healing; to fast for belief in yourself; to fast for physical, mental, and emotional strength; to fast for hope during hard times; and to fast for wholeness to become the person God created you to be.

Once you can control your physical desires and human short-comings, you will realize just how powerful God has created you to be. Your faith will flourish. You will be able to stand in your power as a child of the highest God, who created you in His image. He sent Jesus Christ to live among us and show us how to live. He even gave up His Son as the ultimate act of uncon-ditional love, showing us that we are made new in His love and forgiveness.

Fasting is a beautiful way to connect with God and show Him that you trust the body He created for you.

How amazing is it that, as a surgeon, I can cut you open— through your skin, your fascia, the muscle of your uterus— pull your baby out, then put some sutures in to put those tissues next to each other, and they will heal back together? The sutures don't heal you, they simply keep the tissue in close approximation, so your body can do its magic (using its innate intelligence) and grow those tissues back together!

No medicine or doctor in the world can do what your body can do through God's creation. Marvel in that understanding for a moment.

Our bodies have an amazing innate intelligence.

You've heard of emotional intelligence? Our body has cellular intelligence, too. I'm going to show you how to activate it.

Create in me a clean heart, O God, and renew a right spirit within me.

−Psalm 51:10

Chapter 3

Find Your Lost Intuition

When I was a little girl, I could tell which grown-ups I could trust just by listening to my gut—that was my intuition. Why do we say we feel it in our gut? Because our gut has an extra nervous system, beyond our central nervous system, called the enteric nervous system. It responds to physical signals from our stomach (like food needing to be digested) by producing chemicals to send signals elsewhere and physically moving the organs of our digestive tract. But even more amazing, it creates chemicals in response to our thoughts (often subconscious ones) and feelings. That is how we can get an "upset stomach" when our intuition is telling us to beware ("that person is sketchy") or we are afraid or stewing over something that is concerning us.

Sometimes the enteric nervous system, along with our central nervous system, gets chronically overactive because we are stuck in fear-based patterns of thinking and being. As a collective society, we chronically feel stressed because we are afraid of failing, not living up to a certain set of standards, not being accepted by others, or not being seen as good enough, smart enough, or competent. This often manifests as gut symptoms; we call irritable bowel syndrome (IBS).

I had IBS for 20 years. We say we "have it," like it is something we catch, when in reality it's a made-up name given to the situation of our nervous system being overly stimulated and stuck. The energy and signals can't flow freely back and forth. Our thoughts and our feelings have gotten away from us, and our bodies have become disconnected from our soul. This can present as a symptom of diarrhea, constipation, upset stomach, or cramping. For others, ignoring our intuition can present differently, such as anxiety, loneliness, or obesity.

Your soul is directly connected to your physical body. Don't believe me?

Watch the mother whose child is hospitalized or the man whose wife just died and see how they function. They can't eat, they can't sleep, they can't think straight, and they are often diagnosed with a chronic illness, like cancer, 6-12 months later. The pain your soul feels absolutely gets translated into your cells and affects how they function.

This connection and communication are bidirectional. We are constantly receiving input from our soul into our physical body and our physical body is constantly sending back messages/signals to our soul.

Our soul is trying to tell us something really important, but we have disconnected our body and soul. We have also disconnected from our intuition; from the Holy Spirit. I believe God talks to our soul through the Holy Spirit and it's our job to be open to receiving those messages. Those messages often come as physical discomfort. This is how the rest of the animal kingdom functions—they receive danger signals and respond accordingly. Unfortunately, we have become conditioned to ignore those messages or cover them up. We learn to tune God out. We learn to cover up those symptoms with band-aids—in my case it was with Pepto-Bismol, Tums, and prescription medications.

Please understand that symptoms are not only a message from your body, but also from God. He is trying to tell you to pay attention because something isn't right.

For me, my body was trying to tell me that my soul was lonely and lost. The Holy Spirit was trying to wake me up to the fact that I wasn't living into my purpose. I was going through the motions of life and not listening to what my heart and soul were longing for. This presented as IBS. I spent years in misery trying to fix my body medically, when in reality, it was my soul that needed healing. I needed to realign my body with my mind and my soul.

As soon as I started feeding my soul by reading the living, breathing Word of the Bible, listening to worship music, going to church regularly, and living as Christ's hands to serve, my body started to truly heal and function the way it was meant to once again. The amazing part? You can always begin again. That is how graceful our God is. He sent His only Son, Jesus Christ, to pay for our sins, our errors, our shortcomings, so we don't have to live in regret or despair. You can simply choose to forgive yourself for not taking care of your body consistently and begin again.

I believe our intuition is the Holy Spirit speaking to our soul. It signals the innate intelligence in our bodies to pay attention and respond. It wants to guide us back to God; He wants us to rely on Him.

It is equally important to understand that we must, as Christians, practice discernment. We must take the time to become mindful and be in constant conversion with God and know His Word, so we know it is Him who is sending these messages.

> *Dear friends, do not believe every spirit, but test the spirits to see whether they are from God, because many false prophets have gone out into the world.*
>
> *–1 John 4*

First and foremost, we are souls created by God having a physical earthly experience. We must remember that we have been given the gift of being guided by the Holy Spirit through our savior Jesus Christ. We have been called to live a life greater than the physical realm. It is our job to continually fight against the complacency of just being human, just focusing on the physical realm, and being persuaded by the darkness.

God taught us the superpower of fasting when He left Jesus in the desert for 40 days and 40 nights to be tempted by evil spirits and earthly ways. Jesus showed us how fasting can draw us closer to God. Fasting is a way to gain control of our physical bodies, quiet the noise from the darkness and physical realm, and develop our discernment. Fasting teaches us that we are greater than our physical desires and that our soul should be leading the decisions in our life. Unfortunately, for many of us, we allow our bodies or dark influences to make daily decisions about our life. Learning to fast is the quickest, most powerful way to flip this around to strengthen our spiritual connection and grow our soul.

That is why it's imperative that you feed your soul by fasting your body.

> *For our struggle is not against flesh and blood, but against the rulers, against the authorities, against the powers of this dark world and against the spiritual forces of evil in the heavenly realms.*
>
> *–Ephesians 6:12*

Cellular intelligence

"Your body has natural healing capacities that nobody in the field of medicine can pretend ultimately to understand."

–Wayne Dyer

I remember being diagnosed with IBS during my first year of medical school. Every time I had to take an exam, which was two to three times every week, I ended up running to the bathroom with stomach cramps and diarrhea. Then I would be constipated and not have a bowel movement for a few days until it was time for the next exam. This vicious cycle got worse as time went on.

I remember being on a four-week rotation with a breast surgeon in the office. I had to go in and talk to a patient before the doctor did—that was how we practiced and learned how to interview patients. There I was, a fresh 26-year-old woman, listening to a 50-year-old woman telling me through her tears and a broken voice how she was just diagnosed with cancer and had to have her breasts removed. Instead of being fully present in the moment and empathizing with her, I was praying to God to stop the cramping inside of me and to be able to hold my bowels long enough to get through that interaction. As soon as she paused and stopped crying, I excused myself, ran to the bathroom, and had explosive diarrhea. That was a mortifying experience and worse yet, nothing I was learning in medical school was helping me figure out what was wrong with me.

IBS was a newer diagnosis in medicine in 2001, even though it has been described in writings as far back as the 1820s. IBS is a common disorder characterized by irregular bowel habits often associated with discomfort. The diagnosis IBS was essentially created because patients were having a constellation of symptoms that couldn't be explained on a physical exam, through endoscopy, or imaging.

Even though the medical community admits that IBS seems to be triggered by stress, they haven't focused on how to decrease stress or heal the gut as a treatment. To this day, the conventional medical community continues to ignore the thousands of studies and research articles linking gut dysbiosis from our SAD to IBS. They focus on prescribing drugs that either slow down or speed up your intestines to stop the symptoms of diarrhea and constipation. Unfortunately, those drugs come with terrible side effects and as soon as you stop them, the problem returns with a vengeance.

IBS is a functional problem at the microscopic level that is intricately directed by our nervous system, but also by bad bacteria running the show and therefore the function of digesting, assimilating, absorbing food, and excreting waste is disrupted. Unfortunately, not recognizing gut dysbiosis as the root cause prevents your doctor from being able to actually treat the condition and get you back to normal function and health.

IBS often leads to hormone imbalances for reasons that I will explain in the coming chapters. It is imperative that you get your microbiome balanced if you want to get your hormones balanced and actually cure your gynecological conditions.

For example, we now understand that certain bacteria in an imbalanced ratio affect our weight. A high amount of Firmicutes living in the gut and low amount of Bacteroidetes (resulting in a high F/B ratio) suggest microbial imbalance, which may be related to increased caloric extraction from food, fat deposition and lipogenesis, impaired insulin sensitivity, and increased inflammation. That is scientific talk that really means that the type of bacteria living in your gut can be a cause of you gaining weight.

Let's talk DNA

Functional medicine reminded me that our bodies have an amazing innate intelligence. Our cells are continually talking to each other and informing one another of their struggles and needs by way of chemical messengers, hormones, neurotransmitters, and protein synthesis from reading our DNA. This means our immune system talks to our hormones, our gut talks to our brain, our adrenal glands talk to our gut, etc.

What's even more amazing? Our cells also talk to our microbiomes—the trillions of bacteria, yeast, viruses, and parasites that cohabitate in and on our bodies. We are actually composed of more bacterial DNA than human DNA! Our gut microbiome alone weighs three to four pounds. Just because you can't see each bacterium individually doesn't mean it's not there. I find that fascinating. They really are "running the show" when it comes to our bodies' functioning.

As soon as we are born, we become colonized from the bacteria that was living in our mother's vaginal tract; hopefully she passed down beneficial microbes like Lactobacillus.

Babies delivered via cesarean section and those not exclusively breastfed, however, may be colonized by skin and hospital-acquired bacteria, such as Staphylococcus and Acinetobacter, leading to a microbiome that is initially less diverse and less healthy. These infants seem more susceptible to developing asthma, allergic rhinitis, diabetes, and coeliac disease.[8]

Our gut microbiome is responsible for so many essential functions. They synthesize our B vitamins and vitamin K. They produce short-chain fatty acids, necessary for a healthy gut. They digest our food into absorbable amino acids (from protein), vitamins, minerals, sugars (from carbohydrates), and lipids (from

---

[8] Sidhu M, van der Poorten D. The gut microbiome. Aust Fam Physician. 2017;46(4):206-211. PMID: 28376573.

fats). They produce neurotransmitters or their precursors, including serotonin, tryptophan, gamma-aminobutyric acid (GABA), dopamine, l-dopa, and noradrenaline. These neurotransmitters communicate with the central nervous system through multiple pathways, including the vagus nerve and the HPA (hypothalamic–pituitary-adrenal) axis.

The gut microbiome also helps produce cortisol, ghrelin, leptin, and glucagon-like peptide. These hormones regulate our feelings of hunger and fullness, which means that our microbiome affects our eating habits. Incredible!

Good guys/Bad guys

A healthy gut has mostly beneficial bacteria (good guys) and not too many opportunistic bacteria, pathogens, yeast, parasites, viruses, or worms (these are all bad guys). Too often we develop gut dysbiosis. This describes the imbalance of too many bad guys and not enough good guys. Bad bacteria often produce gas (like methane) as a by-product, giving the symptom of gas and bloating. They often produce lipopolysaccharides (LPS), which is a toxin that seeps into our bloodstream and causes inflammation, showing up as joint pain, brain fog, headaches, and insomnia.

I'm going to teach you that when and what we eat determines what lives and thrives in our gut and controls how our body functions.

There are beneficial bacteria, like Akkermansia and Faecalibacterium, that grow and thrive from God's food. These bacteria produce a mucosal barrier over the single layer of epithelial cells that line the gut. These cells are the gate-keeper of what enters our blood stream and what doesn't. This barrier helps prevent unwanted and dangerous toxins, undigested foods, parasites, and foreign materials from entering into our body. In other words, our gut microbiome is necessary for protection from the outside world. I will explain this in more detail in Chapter 5 and how it relates to our immune system. God knew all the dangers we would encounter, and He equipped us to combat it, but it's our job to understand and nurture that process.

Our microbiome also assists our immune system. An incredible 70-80% of our immune system is our gut. That goes to show how important the ecosystem of our gut really is! God created us to co-exist with completely different species, living inside of us through our entire lives. This ecosystem has its own cellular intelligence and signaling system, which is way beyond the scope of this book. But it bears mentioning because God's creations are beyond our wildest imaginations and I would encourage you to be a life-long learner. Get curious. Keep searching for a deeper understanding of how you—not only the physical you, but also the spiritual you—fit into this incredible greater gift we call life.

In Chapter 5 we'll dive deeper into our immune system because it is a huge missing piece of the puzzle when trying to figure out why our body isn't functioning the way we want it, whether that is with not being able to lose weight or have energy, or be free from symptoms, like migraines.

Before we go there, we have to talk about willpower and cravings. Do you wonder why willpower isn't enough to stop you from eating Frankenfoods? Or maybe you're saying, "I eat clean and don't have a sweet tooth, so what's wrong with me?"

Whatever your specific question or concern is, I'm going to address it. Stick with me!

For everything in the world—the lust of the flesh, the lust of the eyes, and the pride of life—comes not from the Father but from the world. - 1 John 2:16

Chapter 4

Truth Behind Cravings

Beat the cravings

For me, cravings from those Frankenfoods were my downfall. This was most evident when I ate gluten (the protein found in wheat). For many people like me, when we digest gluten, our body produces peptides called gluteomorphins, which act on the same receptors as morphine. This causes a mild feeling of euphoria, like when you take the pain killer morphine. It makes you feel really good, and when it's gone, you crave it again. You want that feeling back.

I was addicted to gluten from a young age. I remember eating a bowl of cereal, only to go back 20 minutes later and eat another bowl because I didn't feel satisfied. I would make "sugar sandwiches," which was me simply pouring white sugar onto a piece of bread, folding it in half and eating it. I even went on to teach my siblings my bad habits.

When I was nine years old, my little sister was born. At 11, my brother came along. At 14, another little sister joined us. I spent many Saturdays babysitting them while my parents worked. Every weekend I would pull out the fryer, the can of Crisco, and a couple tubes of ready-to-bake biscuits. I would use the cap from a two-liter bottle to cut a hole in the middle of the biscuit to make homemade donuts and donut holes. Once the Crisco was spitting, I would drop them in the fryer until they turned a golden brown, pull them out, put them into a brown bag full of cinnamon and sugar, and shake them until they were perfect. As soon as my brother and sisters heard the bag shaking, they would run into the kitchen all excited, jumping up and down. It was the best part of our day. My mouth waters just thinking about how yummy they were. The problem was, I would eat an entire can by myself and still want more.

This way of eating only magnified as I aged. I lived on ramen noodles, mac 'n' cheese, and pizza. Gluten and sugar talked to me. Eventually I learned that those gluteomorphins and sugar-highs gave me a temporary good feeling that washed away bad feelings. I learned how to use food as my emotional regulator. When I was sad or lonely, I ate; when I was stressed, I ate; when I was bored, I ate. Even once I became an attending physician, I still ate like a teenager. I still ate to control my feelings. This wasn't anything I was aware of until recently.

There I was, 40 years old, board-certified in obstetrics and gynecology, chief of the OB department, a highly accomplished robotic surgeon, performing complicated cases for severe endometriosis, fibroids, and other benign tumors, trying to help women feel better when secretly I felt just as miserable as they did.

On my office days when I was seeing patients all day, doing pap smears, annual exams, colposcopies, watching women in labor, etc., I would be distracted by thoughts of the bagels or donuts

in the breakroom. (I swear every week we were celebrating someone's birthday because there was always cake in the breakroom.
Can you relate?) I ate those things from the minute I walked into
the office at 7am, every couple of hours, until I left at 6 or 7pm
each night. If I tried to abstain then I couldn't function. I always
gave in, just to stop the cravings.

I know now that isn't how God wanted me to live.

Are you struggling with cravings?

Sugar is now in almost everything we consume, so we don't
even realize we are addicted. In the 1800s, Americans consumed
two pounds of sugar per person per year. Today we average 60
pounds per person per year! According to the AHA, women
should only get 10% of their calories from sugar. That would
be six teaspoons per day (or 25 grams). For reference: One can
of soda (or pop if you're from Michigan, like me) contains eight
teaspoons (32 grams) of added sugar![9] We are exceeding our
daily limit with one beverage.

Currently, we consume over a pound of sugar *per week*! Those
numbers are astonishing, but because it's been slowly invading
the food industry over decades, we don't realize just how much
we're consuming. We have gotten to the point where we think
drinking 65 grams of sugar disguised as our morning coffee is
okay because we all do it.

The cereal/breakfast industry has duped us into eating nothing but sugar for breakfast disguised as bagels, muffins, cereal,
oatmeal, and bars. That is the absolute worst way to start your
day because it puts you on the sugar rollercoaster for the rest
of the day. As soon as your sugar level drops, you want more to
level out the roller coaster.

The only way to stop the madness and resulting weight gain,
brain fog, "hangry" episodes, chronic inflammation, and disease

---

[9] "How much sugar is too much?" American Heart Association, Inc. (Online
     Resource)

processes from setting in is to stop riding the sugar roller coaster. When we eat every few hours, even if it's a handful of almonds, a cheese stick, or a few M&Ms, we are getting back on the roller coaster. We keep topping off our blood sugar. As soon as it starts to decrease, we eat something (usually carbohydrates) and that increases our levels again.

Our pancreas has to work non-stop to make insulin, which is a fat-storage hormone. Insulin goes and transports the glucose (sugar) out of the blood into the cells. If we aren't physically using that glucose for energy, our body will convert it into fat and store it for later. This is why we are seeing more and more people developing fatty liver. We are eating way too much sugar and way too many carbohydrates and our body doesn't know where to put it all.

The SAD diet is destroying us!

For decades the snacking industry has brainwashed us into thinking that fat makes us fat. They created all kinds of Franken-foods with fake fats called "trans fats" to deceive us and make us believe those processed foods weren't harming us. When they made these low-fat and no-fat "foods," they quickly realized that they needed to add lots of sugar and other flavorings to make it taste good and create ever-lasting cravings so people would want to continue consuming their products. This is how we went from ingesting two pounds of sugar per person per year to 60 pounds per year.

We now know the truth: Fat doesn't make us fat; sugar makes us fat!

Cholesterol is not the villain

It took almost 20 years of the low-fat, no-fat diet wreaking havoc on our systems for conventional cardiology to finally admit they were wrong. And guess who was driving this narrative the whole time? The Frankenfood industry. They have way more control over how medicine is practiced in this country than even the doctors realize. I know I didn't realize it when I was stuck in that broken system. Some of the most prestigious hospitals in the country have Little Caesars, Coke, McDonalds, and Starbucks in their cafeteria. Those "foods" are not healthy. They have clearly been linked to disease, yet we promote them as harmless and deny their effect on our health.

And can we please talk about cholesterol? Cholesterol should not be feared. It does not cause disease. Inflammation causes disease. So, then why did cholesterol get the blame?

Because cholesterol was there at the scene. Imagine someone has a heart attack. Doctors look at the coronary arteries feeding blood to the heart muscle. They see plagues of cholesterol partially blocking the artery. They assumed that person had too much cholesterol and so it was getting stuck in the arteries, causing a blockage of blood flow, leading to a heart attack. This theory was accepted and not questioned and debunked until the late 1990s.[10,11,12,13] Unfortunately, the damage of perpetuating this untruth prevails to this day.

We now understand that there is underlying inflammation, usually stemming from gut dysbiosis, intestinal permeability

[10]   Adams DD. The great cholesterol myth; unfortunate consequences of Brown and Goldstein's mistake. QJM. 2011 Oct;104(10):867-70. doi: 10.1093/qjmed/hcr087. Epub 2011 Jun 20. PMID: 21690178.
[11]   Tsoupras A, Lordan R, Zabetakis I. Inflammation, not Cholesterol, Is a Cause of Chronic Disease. Nutrients. 2018 May 12;10(5):604. doi: 10.3390/nu10050604. PMID: 29757226; PMCID: PMC5986484.
[12]   Yusuf S, Hawken S, Ounpuu S, Dans T, Avezum A, Lanas F, McQueen M, Budaj A, Pais P, Varigos J, Lisheng L; INTERHEART Study Investigators. Effect of potentially modifiable risk factors associated with myocardial infarction in 52 countries (the INTERHEART study): case-control study. Lancet. 2004 Sep 11-17;364(9438):937-52. doi: 10.1016/S0140-6736(04)17018-9. PMID: 15364185.
[13]   Alston MC, Redman LM, Sones JL. An Overview of Obesity, Cholesterol, and Systemic Inflammation in Preeclampsia. Nutrients. 2022 May 17;14(10):2087. doi: 10.3390/nu14102087. PMID: 35631228; PMCID: PMC9143481.

"leaky gut," or environmental exposures, driving these processes. Those toxins cause microscopic damage to the artery wall, then cholesterol, calcium, and other repair chemicals go to the "scene of the crime" and try to repair the damage. Cholesterol is actually trying to repair the situation, but because the initial inflammatory trigger isn't usually removed (the root cause), then the artery can't heal and the process worsens despite cholesterol's best efforts.

Unfortunately, the American Heart Association (AHA), the food industry, medical schools, the pharmaceutical industry, and doctors (especially cardiologists), have all inadvertently affected women's hormones with their terrible dietary restrictions and recommendations and their excess prescribing of statin medications. A statin is a medication designed to decrease your cholesterol level. Atorvastatin (brand name, Lipitor) is the most prescribed drug in the U.S. In 2019, it was prescribed to 24.5 million people.[14] Pfizer makes $2 billion (yes billion with a "b") every year from this one drug.[15]

Cholesterol is actually the backbone ingredient to making your sex hormones—progesterone, estrogen, DHEA, and testosterone. It's also required for healthy cell membranes (remember how your body is made of trillions of cells?) where your hormone receptors are. Receptors are the lock and your hormones are the key.

You can't make hormones and hormones can't send their signals without cholesterol! Please don't be afraid of cholesterol.

---

14   "Ranked: The Most Prescribed Drugs in the U.S." by Omri Wallach, November 1, 2021. Visual Capitalist. (Online Article)

15   "Lipitor is still churning out billions of dollars," by Bob Herman, Oct 30, 2019. Axios. (Online Article)

Sugar is toxic

So how does sugar make us fat?

When you eat sugar—whether it's in the form of table sugar, orange juice, honey, strawberries, grapes, bread, crackers, quinoa, or gummy bears—it gets broken down into its main chemical components in the stomach and small intestine. Once the sugar is broken down into its components, those molecules get absorbed into the bloodstream.

The word "sugar" often refers to any carbohydrate. Carbohydrates are a bunch of sugar molecules all connected. Simple sugars are called monosaccharides and include glucose, fructose, and galactose. Compound sugars, also called disaccharides (meaning two sugars), are molecules made of two connected monosaccharides; examples are sucrose (glucose + fructose), lactose (glucose + galactose), and maltose (two molecules of glucose). White table sugar is a refined form of sucrose. Longer chains of sugar are called oligosaccharides and polysaccharides. Starch is a form of multiple glucoses chained together and is found in plants.

In the body, these compound sugars are broken down into the simple sugars. Sugars are found in the tissues of most plants. Fruits and honey are natural sources of simple sugars. Maltose is produced by malting grain. Interestingly, lactose is the only sugar that isn't extracted from plants. It can only be found in milk and dairy products, and is abundant in human breast milk.

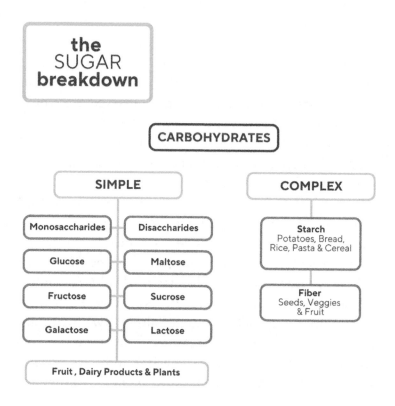

The food and snacking industry eventually developed corn syrup, which is a cheaper source of sugar. They take the starch of the corn, which gets broken into simple sugars, such as maltose, fructose, and glucose and turn it into corn syrup. High fructose corn syrup has been one of the biggest culprits to create inflammation, chronic disease, and tooth decay. Part of the reason is because they use genetically modified corn, which causes destruction of the cells in our gut (aka leaky gut). This creation has forever changed us as a civilization. Corn syrup is used as a sweetener and thickening agent for almost all processed foods today.

Read your labels. It's in salad dressings, ketchup, health bars, cereal, pop/soda, yogurt, baked goods, canned soups and fruits, teas, coffee drinks, and the list goes on and on.

When we consume sugar or its polysaccharide versions, our body breaks it down and absorbs it into our bloodstream. Then our body either has to use that sugar to create ATP (energy) or it has to store it for later use. The body doesn't like too much sugar in the bloodstream because it changes the pH and osmolarity of the blood. The blood is tightly regulated, so your body is always surveilling your blood sugar levels and producing insulin in response to those levels.

Because of this innate cellular level intelligence, our bodies have an amazing ability to maintain homeostasis. For example, it keeps our blood in a specific pH range of 7.40. Regulation of body fluid pH is one of the most important physiological functions of homeostasis, because activity of most chemical reactions via enzyme proteins is dependent on proper fluid pH.[16]

If our body suffers enough insult, that homeostasis (balance) will be disrupted and disease will develop, like insulin resistance, hypertension, and visceral obesity (ya know, the fat that you can't suck in... You feel bloated and look five months pregnant all the time).

When our blood sugar (glucose) is elevated (from our diet of boxed and bagged foods or from our chronic stress-filled lives), it signals our pancreas to produce and secrete insulin. Insulin then takes the glucose out of our blood stream and moves it to the liver to be utilized as energy or stored as fat. Insulin is a fat-storing hormone.

---

[16] Aoi W, Marunaka Y. Importance of pH homeostasis in metabolic health and diseases: crucial role of membrane proton transport. Biomed Res Int. 2014;2014:598986. doi: 10.1155/2014/598986. Epub 2014 Sep 11. PMID: 25302301; PMCID: PMC4180894.

If our blood sugar is constantly elevated and insulin is constantly having to transfer and store the glucose, our cells get tired of insulin knocking on the door, saying, "Let in the sugar. Please store more sugar."

Your body must then produce more insulin to send the same signal because the cells are becoming deaf; they don't want to listen.

This is known as insulin resistance.

If this continues, you eventually develop diabetes. Diabetes is the result of chronically elevated blood sugar that requires more and more insulin to handle it, eventually resulting in our pancreas being unable to keep up with the demands of producing so much insulin.

Obesity epidemic

This blood sugar issue often presents itself in women over age 45, but we're seeing it in younger women now. This is the main issue with polycystic ovarian syndrome (PCOS) as well. Women (and the same is true for men) start waking up during the night to urinate. This is often a blood sugar problem, but most conventional doctors will blame menopause or a weak bladder and dismiss a woman's concerns, so the issue goes unaddressed and eventually leads to insulin resistance and diabetes.

Please understand, conventional doctors are trained to look for a disease diagnosis and then come up with a medication or surgical procedure to "fix it." I call this band-aid medicine because it's focused on treating symptoms and managing disease; it's not asking why or addressing the root cause issue. It's also not looking at trends and trying to reverse disease processes that are beginning.

For example, if you see your conventional doctor, they will check your fasting blood sugar and if it's less than 120, they will tell you you're fine and to return in a year. (I know because this is how I was trained and encouraged to practice for over a decade.) They might draw a HgbA1c (which is a marker for your average blood sugar over a three-month time period) and if it's less than 6%, they will tell you that you are fine. I say "might" because insurance often dictates how physicians/practitioners practice medicine. Usually, insurance won't cover a HgbA1c unless you already have a diagnosis of diabetes, so most doctors and other practitioners won't order it.

If you see a functional medicine practitioner like myself, he or she will evaluate your HgbA1c and fasting insulin over time to look for trends. If that practitioner sees that you are on the path toward developing insulin resistance or diabetes, we can intervene to turn things around and get you on a different path, instead of waiting until your body has gone off the cliff and you have diabetes that requires medication potentially for the rest of your life.

If your HgbA1c is 5.6%, I'm going to tell you that you are on the path toward prediabetes and we need to intervene so you don't continue down that path. I am also going to check a fasting insulin level to see how your pancreas is responding with insulin production. This will give me a better picture of how aggressive we need to be to turn things around.

A conventional physician will tell you that a HgbA1c of 5.6% is fine and to return in a year. Sadly, that following year, you will most likely have prediabetes.

A conventional physician may recommend that you "eat less and exercise more," which is terrible advice (as you'll soon find out why), or they may recommend you to "eat healthier," but they most likely won't give you any clear guidance on how to do that.

That's one reason I wrote this book!

Within three to five years, most patients will have gone on to develop diabetes.[17] That's when the doctor intervenes. You will be prescribed medication like metformin pills or semaglutide injections. You will have to check your blood sugar regularly to see if you need your medication adjusted. And you will be at an increased risk of all the diseases that are associated with that, including hypertension, heart disease, nerve damage, loss of sexual function, and Alzheimer's.

The statistics on diabetes are startling. According to the CDC:[18]

- 37.3 million people have diabetes

- 8.5 million people are undiagnosed

- 96 million people aged 18 years or older have prediabetes (38% of the adult U.S. population).

Could you have fatty liver?

Just as concerning as diabetes is the rise in non-alcoholic fatty liver disease (NAFLD). It is now the most common liver disease in the world and may soon become the most common indication for liver transplantation.[19] According to the National Institute of Health (NIH), 24% of U.S. adults and 5-10% of children have developed fatty liver![20]

---

[17] About Prediabetes and Type 2 Diabetes. Centers for Disease Control and Prevention (Online Resource)

[18] National Diabetes Statistics Report. Centers for Disease Control and Prevention (Online Resource)

[19] Perumpail BJ, Khan MA, Yoo ER, Cholankeril G, Kim D, Ahmed A. Clinical epidemiology and disease burden of nonalcoholic fatty liver disease. World J Gastroenterol. 2017 Dec 21;23(47):8263-8276. doi: 10.3748/wjg.v23.i47.8263. PMID: 29307986; PMCID: PMC5743497.

[20] Nonalcoholic Fatty Liver Disease (NAFLD) & NASH. National Institute of Diabetes and Digestive and Kidney Diseases (NIDDK), U.S. Department of Health and Human Services, and National Institutes of Health (Online Resource)

Once we have fatty liver, our liver struggles to do its normal detox processes, like metabolizing our hormones or inactivating toxins or medications that we've ingested. It also struggles to make necessary proteins like ferritin, which carries iron and vitamin K, which are necessary for blood clotting and converting our inactive T4 thyroid hormone into active T3 hormone. This has contributed to a rise in women being diagnosed with hypothyroidism. You can imagine how systemic and wide-spread the effects of fatty liver can be on a person's health.

Sugar and simple carbohydrates can also cause candida (aka yeast or fungal) overgrowth in our gut. When the yeast consumes the sugars we ingest, it produces alcohol (ethanol) and acetaldehyde (this is the chemical responsible for the main symptoms of a hangover) as a byproduct.[21,22] This gives us brain fog, fatigue, and other symptoms. The yeast wants to survive, so it sends signals to your brain and contributes to your cravings. It's important to starve them off.

And why is all this happening? Because we are consuming way too much sugar and simple carbohydrates, and we are eating both of those way too often. All these behaviors change our gut microbiome for the worse and they contribute to the problem as well.

That means it's time to break up with sugar!

How do we prevent this or reverse this if it's already happened? We change what and how we are eating. We fast!

---

[21]   Mbaye B, Borentain P, Magdy Wasfy R, Alou MT, Armstrong N, Mottola G, Meddeb L, Ranque S, Gérolami R, Million M, Raoult D. Endogenous Ethanol and Triglyceride Production by Gut Pichia kudriavzevii, Candida albicans and Candida glabrata Yeasts in Non-Alcoholic Steatohepatitis. Cells. 2022 Oct 27;11(21):3390. doi: 10.3390/cells11213390. PMID: 36359786; PMCID: PMC9654979.

[22]   Bayoumy AB, Mulder CJJ, Mol JJ, Tushuizen ME. Gut fermentation syndrome: A systematic review of case reports. United European Gastroenterol J. 2021 Apr;9(3):332-342. doi: 10.1002/ueg2.12062. Epub 2021 Apr 22. PMID: 33887125; PMCID: PMC8259373.

What happens in fat cells?

Another important factor contributing to us holding onto excess weight and developing these diseases is toxins in our environment. Thousands of chemicals have been created in a lab—chemicals that didn't exist just 100 years ago.[23] Since the beginning of time, the human body has had to handle toxins coming into the body, like spoiled meat with bad bacteria, contaminated water with parasites, and poisonous plants, mushrooms, and berries. God created our bodies with detoxification mechanisms and an immune system to handle all those insults. But this last century's creations have bombarded our bodies with foreign, never-before-seen toxins that man created. Our bodies are working overtime to combat these, but are losing the battle because we aren't intervening and giving the body what it needs.

One of the most abundant and toxic chemicals is plastics because the majority of them never disintegrate, hence why they are called forever toxins. Worse yet, these plastics act as xenoestrogens (aka endocrine disruptors).[24] These are chemicals in the environment that get into our body, bind to our estrogen receptors, and send the same signals that estrogen would send. Estrogen is our main reproductive growth hormone, so these toxic chemicals can contribute to PMS, heavy periods, fibrocystic breasts, uterine fibroids, endometriosis, and other hormone imbalances, which is why it's super important to actively decrease your exposure to them.

---

[23] "The public health impact of chemicals: knowns and unknowns," 23 May 2016. World Health Organization (Online Article).

[24] Paterni I, Granchi C, Minutolo F. Risks and benefits related to alimentary exposure to xenoestrogens. Crit Rev Food Sci Nutr. 2017 Nov 2;57(16):3384-3404. doi: 10.1080/10408398.2015.1126547. PMID: 26744831; PMCID: PMC6104637.

Want more info? Please scan the QR code for my short e-guide: *How to Decrease Your Toxic Burden.*

Xenoestrogens are common in plastics, perfumes, lotions, candles, and beauty products. They are chemicals like BPA (bisphenol A), phthalates, parabens, etc. Because they have only recently been introduced into our world, our great-grand-mothers and ancestors were never exposed to such things. Their bodies never had to try to detox these foreign compounds. Now, our bodies are struggling to survive in a world full of foreign chemicals that they weren't designed to deal with. Once these chemicals get in our bodies, our liver doesn't know how to handle them, so most of it gets stored in our fat cells, in an effort to protect our vital organs (like our brain, heart, and kidneys). The more xenoestrogens we absorb, the more fat cells we need to store them.

And what happens in fat cells? Estrone is made. Estrone is a form of estrogen that we don't want too much of because its metabolite, or breakdown product, can cause a quinone reaction, which damages cells and increases your risk of developing breast and uterine cancer. This increased estrone causes our fat cells to be more metabolically active, so we can store more xenoestrogens in the fat in an effort to protect our vital organs from these xenoestrogens. The whole process gets us stuck in a vicious cycle of weight gain. And when you try to lose weight, your body resists because it doesn't want to put those toxins back into your bloodstream, so you develop weight loss resistance in an effort to protect yourself.

These environmental xenoestrogens are a big reason why certain forms of cancer have dramatically increased over the past 40 years. It's not the hormones our body makes that we need to be concerned about, it's the synthetic "hormone-like compounds" that we are eating, drinking, breathing, and absorbing through our skin that create hormone imbalances and have contributed to a sharp rise in obesity in not only women, but men and children as well. This is a big reason we are seeing puberty at a younger age, men with "man boobs," and weight gain more in a female distribution pattern around the hips and thighs, as well as a huge increase in infertility.

According to the CDC, at least 20% of the 72 million women ages 15-49 ingest (as a pill) or absorb (as an injection, implant, or IUD) synthetic hormones for birth control.[25] These man-made hormones are also xenoestrogens. Women metabolize then urinate these xenoestrogens every single day into our environment. Those xenoestrogens have infiltrated our water supply and soil in levels that, I can only imagine, are drastically high, because they haven't been tested or investigated. I find that very concerning.

Please don't misunderstand my intention in mentioning these things. I am all for empowering women to have control over their reproductive abilities. I would not have been able to go back and get my GED, get through college and medical school had I not had birth control to prevent another pregnancy. However, I do believe we should know what we are signing up for and understand the bigger impact this has on our society, environment, and health as a whole. These things need to be

---

[25]   Current Contraceptive Status Among Women Aged 15–49: United States, 2015–2017. Kimberly Daniels, Ph.D., and Joyce C. Abma, Ph.D. NCHS Data Brief No. 327, December 2018. Centers for Disease Control and Prevention (Online Article)

addressed. For more understanding of the impact birth control has on our health, I invite you to listen to my podcast, *The Gutsy Gynecologist Show*, or watch it on YouTube, where I discuss these topics and all things impacting women's health.

As you can see, it's more important than ever to decrease your exposure going forward and to remove the toxins you already have stored in order to break through weight loss resistance.

The culmination of these toxic chemicals and the SAD diet causes wide-spread chronic inflammation, and this is the basis for almost all modern diseases like obesity, diabetes, heart disease, cancer, autoimmune conditions, and Alzheimer's, to name a few. These diseases didn't exist before we created Frankenfoods and toxic chemicals like plastic. Humans died from viral and bacterial infections or traumatic accidents. Thank goodness modern medicine does exist to often save us from those conditions, but unfortunately, it hasn't figured out how to save us from lifestyle diseases. Thankfully, functional medicine has figured this out, but as of yet, it hasn't been accepted by the greater conventional world.

Frankenfoods cause inflammation

So, what is inflammation? A perfect example of inflammation is when I eat too much sugar, usually in the form of ice cream or candy, my joints flare up in pain.

One weekend, my grandson stayed with us and we had a blast. We ate ice cream three times, had some Halloween candy, and made waffles for breakfast (gluten-free of course). By Monday, my left knee was swollen and throbbing and I could barely walk on it. That knee has been a problem since middle school, but has behaved for years because I was eating clean and avoiding sugar. That weekend of sugar flared it back up!

I hear this from my patients all the time; as soon as they fall off the wagon and eat junk food, their aches and pains come back. Sugar is toxic. It causes inflammation all over your body.

Plant seed oils do the same thing. These are called omega-6 polyunsaturated fats. The most common ones are vegetable, corn, canola, soybean, rapeseed, safflower, sunflower, and cottonseed oils. Please avoid these as much as you possibly can. Once we ingest them, they get converted into arachidonic acid, which causes an inflammatory cascade leading to swelling, joint pain, cellular, and mitochondrial dysfunction.

Instead of seed oils, choose olive, avocado, flaxseed, or coconut oils, or even grass-fed butter. These are higher in omega-3s, which get converted into eicosapentaenoic acid (EPA) and docosahexaenoic acid (DHA), which have anti-inflammatory properties. You might recognize the abbreviations because EPA and DHA are what you get when you take a fish oil supplement.

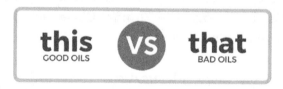

Extra Virgin Olive Oil	Canola & Vegetable Oil
Coconut Oil	Sunflower & Safflower Oil
Avocado Oil	Grapeseed Oil & Corn Oil
Ghee Butter	Cottonseed & Peanut Oil

What drives *your* ailments? Are you addicted to sugar or gluten? Are you consuming omega-6 oils on a regular basis? If so, removing these things is an easy way to start shifting your health.

Now, let's talk about bad advice: Have you ever done cardio until you were blue in the face only to gain weight? Or maybe you've tried counting and cutting calories only to gain weight?

This next section is for you.

"As a functional gynecologist, I never just treat one system because all of our systems work together to create the body we are living in. And I never just treat the physical body because the health of our mind and soul equally impacts our body's ability to thrive."

–Dr. Tabatha

Chapter 5

Change Your Physiology

If you have ever listened to my podcast, *The Gutsy Gynecologist Show*, then you know that I differentiate how I practice medicine now as a functional gynecologist compared to how I practiced as a conventional gynecologist. The way I approach women's diagnoses and symptoms is completely different.

Essentially, a **functional gynecologist** treats the root causes of gynecological issues for resolution of disease as opposed to the conventional band-aid approach of covering up symptoms with medications and surgeries. For example, endometriosis is an inflammatory disease stemming from chronic gut dysbiosis and hormone imbalances.[26,27,28] Unfortunately, **conventional**

26 Elkafas H, Walls M, Al-Hendy A, Ismail N. Gut and genital tract microbiomes: Dysbiosis and link to gynecological disorders. Front Cell Infect Microbiol. 2022 Dec 16;12:1059825. doi: 10.3389/fcimb.2022.1059825. Erratum in: Front Cell Infect Microbiol. 2023 May 12;13:1211349. PMID: 36590579; PMCID: PMC9800796.

27 Jiang I, Yong PJ, Allaire C, Bedaiwy MA. Intricate Connections between the Microbiota and Endometriosis. Int J Mol Sci. 2021 May 26;22(11):5644. doi: 10.3390/ijms22115644. PMID: 34073257; PMCID: PMC8198999.

28 Salliss ME, Farland LV, Mahnert ND, Herbst-Kralovetz MM. The role of gut and genital microbiota and the estrobolome in endometriosis, infertility and chronic pelvic pain. Hum Reprod Update. 2021 Dec 21;28(1):92-131. doi: 10.1093/humupd/dmab035. PMID: 34718567.

gynecologists are not trained to evaluate the gut microbiome for dysbiosis or taught how to balance hormones naturally. We are trained to suppress estrogen production with harsh medications and physically remove endometriosis with advanced surgical techniques.

As a conventionally trained OB/GYN, I also wasn't taught how to stop endometriosis from developing in the first place. I had to learn that through my functional medicine training, which was completely separate from my medical school training, residency, board certification, and menopause certification training. Because I have studied and become certified through many different institutions, I have the unique perspective of understanding both prevention and disease and how providers approach it from different angles, and why the general public is so confused when it comes to women's health advice. That is why I am so passionate to share everything I have learned with you.

I'm about to explain the most common root causes of weight gain and weight loss resistance for women that your conventional doctor isn't telling you about, so keep reading!

Gaining weight from stress

Jen was a 45-year-old woman who went to her primary care physician for weight gain. She had always tried to watch her weight by limiting her fats and choosing diet foods like diet pop and Atkins bars.

She explained, "I don't understand why I'm gaining weight. I used to be able to go on a diet for a month and lose five pounds, but no matter what I try now nothing works."

She mentioned that she had been super stressed at her job and was eating in a rush, often whatever she could find. She was also having trouble falling asleep, so she was drinking wine in the evening to shut her brain off. Of note, she underwent a hysterectomy two years prior for heavy periods.

Her doctor prescribed Adipex (a medication that is supposed to suppress appetite) and Ambien (a medication for sleep). He told her to eat 1,600 calories a day and do cardio workouts three or four times a week. "You just need to burn more calories than you take in. You're obviously eating more than you realize," he told her.

A few months later, Jen scheduled an appointment with me to see if maybe her hormones were the problem.

"I know I've had a hysterectomy and my hormones should be fine, but I'm wondering if my weight issue could be hormonal. I've been taking these medications and can't lose any weight. My brain just seems wired and won't shut off. I fall asleep with the Ambien, but I never feel rested," she told me.

We spent an hour discussing her entire life history and she explained how two years ago she had gone through a terrible divorce and was still feeling bitter about the fact that she had to work so much to pay all the bills.

"It was so stressful. I feel like I'm stuck in hyper-reactive mode," she had said.

I explained to Jen that her stressful divorce forced her body to produce excessive amounts of cortisol and adrenaline on a regular basis for many months.

Cortisol is our main stress hormone that gets released to handle physical stresses like having surgery, running a 5k, or healing a wound. It also gets released when we perceive mental or emotional stress, like feeling afraid or angry.

This chronic overproduction is called adrenal hyperstimulation. Our bodies were originally designed to run from predators (think of cavewomen running from a saber-toothed tiger) and fight off infections; a rush of cortisol helps us do that. Nowadays, we aren't running from tigers, but we are stressing over emails, deadlines, fractured relationships, managing our kids, being disconnected from our Creator, and the stress associated with living lives that aren't truly fulfilling.

Our bodies are also dealing with the chronic physical stress associated with the high load of environmental toxins we are exposed to every day and trying to process those from a physiological standpoint. It is very taxing on our bodies.

When your adrenals glands release cortisol into your bloodstream in response to those stressors, some of it goes to your hypothalamus in your brain. This stimulates corticotropin-releasing hormone (CRH), which goes to your pituitary gland and tells it to make adrenocorticotropic hormone (ACTH), which then goes to your adrenals and tells it to produce more or less cortisol. This communication is called the hypothalamic pituitary adrenal (HPA) axis.

If you continue to ask your body to produce excess cortisol for long periods of time, like Jen did, then your brain will eventually down-regulate your HPA axis in an effort to protect you.

Excess cortisol production from chronic stress is like a mom that keeps yelling louder and louder at her child, day after day, "Pick up your socks, do your homework, stop making a mess!"

Eventually, the child stops listening and learns how to tune out mom's yelling. That results in no socks getting picked up and no homework getting done. Hopefully, at that point the mom realizes her efforts are futile and stops yelling all the time.

This is what happens in your brain. It will stop responding to the cortisol that's yelling louder and louder with more and more cortisol production and eventually learn to tune it out. This is called down-regulation. The brain will stop responding with CRH and ACTH production. This HPA dysfunction will eventually cause your adrenals to stop yelling (making cortisol). This is called stage 3 adrenal dysfunction, which used to be called adrenal fatigue.

In the past it was thought that the adrenal glands stopped being able to physically make cortisol, but we now understand that your body shuts down this production to protect you. It's an example of the incredible innate cellular intelligence I was explaining earlier. Your HPA system essentially goes into survival mode.

This downregulation tells your thyroid that you are now in survival mode and then your thyroid responds accordingly by slowing your metabolism. Why? Because your body perceives that you are in danger, so it wants to conserve energy and not expend more than absolutely necessary.

This is why Jen couldn't lose weight to save her life.

Unfortunately, this scenario is very common and all too often women are advised to eat less and exercise more.

The problem with that?

Calorie restriction and cardio-intense workouts are short-term stressors to the body and require cortisol production, therefore your body perceives this as more stress. The more calorie restriction and cardio workouts, the more HPA axis dysfunction, the more your metabolism slows even further.

From a functional medicine standpoint, I evaluated Jen's physiology with 24-hour saliva cortisol testing and realized that she didn't need an appetite suppressant or a pill to give her false, non-restorative sleep.

She needed to support her HPA axis, so her adrenal glands could go back to producing cortisol in an appropriate 24-hour rhythmic pattern, like they're supposed to.

This required getting control of her "monkey-mind" using guided meditation, prayer, and breathing techniques, setting boundaries with her work schedule, prioritizing self-preservation care every day, doing restorative and muscle-building exercises, eating more healthy fats and clean protein, and working through hurt feelings from her divorce, and creating new thought patterns to stimulate healing.

Regulate your autonomic nervous system

Understanding how to regulate your autonomic nervous system has helped every woman who's ever learned it, so listen up.

God created us to be incredibly resilient. He designed us to survive the most difficult environments imaginable. Because of this, we have two main branches of our nervous system traveling from our brains, down our spinal cord, and out to our organs, innervating every organ, including our muscles and skin: The somatic and autonomic branches. These branches also travel in the opposite direction from the skin and organs back to the brain. The communication is bi-directional.

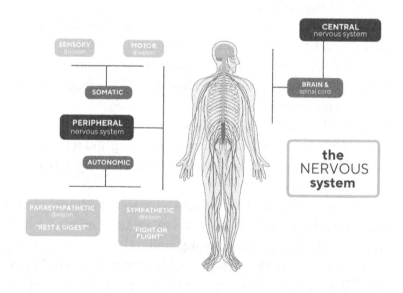

Our somatic branch functions under voluntary input, like when we want to move our arm and then we do so. Conversely, our autonomic nervous system runs all our body's processes without us thinking about it—hence it's automatic.

The autonomic branch tells our lungs to breathe, our intestines to move, our postural muscles to contract and keep us upright, and it tells our adrenal glands when to release cortisol and adrenaline.

The autonomic branch is either in a sympathetic dominant state (fight-or-flight) or in a parasympathetic state (rest-and-digest).

Sympathetic overdrive causes adrenal hyperstimulation, which is what Jen was experiencing for so long.

Unfortunately, your body can't do its parasympathetic jobs very well when the sympathetic system is activated and producing cortisol, adrenaline, and inflammation. This causes symptoms such as weight gain, IBS, brain fog, shortness of breath, panic attacks, heart palpitations, and the inability to fall asleep. This eventually leads to the burn out or the down-regulation I mentioned, which results in chronic fatigue.

The good news? Our bodies have an amazing innate ability to heal and return to homeostasis, *if* we support them.

In Jen's case, we needed to focus on stimulating her parasympathetic nervous system, calming her sympathetic system, and healing all the other systems that were affected.

How chronic stress affects your other systems

Chronic stress and cortisol production causes increased intestinal permeability, aka leaky gut. Leaky gut leads to inflammation throughout your body. How does that happen?

Our intestines have only one cell layer between the lumen (where the food we're digesting and where our gut microbiome lives) and our blood stream; it's called the epithelium.

In between those epithelial cells there are gap junctions that work like doors or toll booths. They open and let in certain things like amino acids, vitamins, and minerals. They close and keep out undigested foods, bacteria, pesticides, viruses, and other foreign invaders. But things break those gap junctions, like too much cortisol (chronic stress), antibiotics, birth control pills and other medications, Frankenfoods, xenoestrogens, and pesticides in our food.

Because our bodies were created with great wisdom, those epithelial cells regenerate every 24-48 hours, but if we have constant insults breaking those gap junctions, things will pass into our bloodstream that should never be there.

Even wiser is the fact that over 70% of our immune system works in our gut, ready to protect us from such a situation. This is the immunoglobulin A (IgA) branch of our immune system, which I will explain more in the next couple pages.

Our immune system is smart enough that it will attack all the things that it doesn't usually see. When it does this, it creates an antibody against that substance, so that any time your body is invaded by that thing again, your immune system knows it's foreign and that it should react.

Unfortunately, in this day and age of huge environmental toxicant overload, our immune systems have had to react more than ever before.

The DNA in your genes (your genetics) hold information with the potential to express certain information. If you have certain genes that make you susceptible to autoimmune diseases (like Hashimoto's thyroiditis, celiac disease, Lupus, or Rheumatoid arthritis), your overactive immune system may activate those genes during an episode of leaky gut.

It isn't guaranteed that those genes will be expressed, but according to the work of Dr. Allesio Fasano, if you have increased intestinal permeability (aka leaky gut) and certain triggers (like Frankenfoods from a poor diet), your immune system will acti-vate those genes and you will develop the autoimmune disease associated with it.

Dr. Fasano is the pioneer behind understanding leaky gut. He has many roles, including being the Director of the Mucosal Immunology and Biology Research Center at MassGeneral hospital for Pediatrics and founding the Center for Celiac Research and Treatment in 1996. In 2000, he and his team discovered the protein zonulin, the major protein released with increased intestinal permeability (aka leaky gut). He has also shown how this plays a role in both inflammation and autoimmunity throughout the body.

Another way your immune system in your gut often over-reacts is by creating antibodies to the "healthy" foods you are eating. Our immune system can create antibodies against foods that aren't themselves inflammatory, but because they were around when your immune system attacked as a response to a leaky gut episode, those foods were attacked; they were shot like innocent bystanders in the line of fire. Now they have an antibody tag against them, so every time you eat that food your immune system says "Oh yeah, we don't like that guy, attack!"

That attack causes an inflammatory cascade reaction, sending cytokines and interleukins into your bloodstream, which contributes to systemic inflammation—the leading driver of chronic diseases like endometriosis, heart disease, diabetes, and Alzheimer's.

Chronic stress and cortisol production also destroys our healthy gut microbiome.

Your gut health determines your gynecologic health

Our microbiome should consist of trillions of diverse bacteria that help us make and absorb vitamins, help us digest our proteins, which help us make neurotransmitters for brain health, help us eliminate our used hormones like estrogen, help remove toxins from the body, and keep bad bacteria, yeast, and parasites from overtaking our digestive tract. Our gut microbiome runs the show. They determine how our body functions.

In Jen's case, we did functional stool testing to evaluate her gut microbiome. It revealed that her chronic stress had killed off her good bacteria. She had yeast overgrowth and some other opportunistic bad bacteria that were producing an enzyme called beta-glucuronidase.

Why was this important to know?

The enzyme beta-glucuronidase is made in small amounts by us, but is produced in larger amounts by bad bacteria. This enzyme essentially cuts the "garbage tag" off your used estrogens that your body is trying to eliminate through your stool. You end up reabsorbing those used estrogens and putting them back into circulation.

Too much estrogen looks like weight gain, irritability, and sleep issues, all which contribute to your stress.

It becomes a vicious cycle!

So why am I telling you this?

Because Jen had to heal her gut in order to repair the damage done by her adrenal dysfunction and get her hormones back into balance.

The functional stool testing and food sensitivity testing we did allowed us to see what exactly was living in her gut and running the show, to see if she was making enough digestive enzymes, to see what her immune system in her gut was doing, and to see whether or not she had active leaky gut that we needed to heal. Zonulin is the protein that is released when those gap junctions get broken between the epithelial cells, so getting a zonulin level on a functional stool test, like GI Map from Diagnostic Solutions, was very helpful in Jen's case.

What I've come to realize is that almost every woman struggling with their hormones benefits from doing gut healing work because hormone imbalance stems from the gut.

The inflammatory cascade

Doing food sensitivity testing with Jen showed us what her immune system was reacting to. It's very common for women to be reacting to many foods if they have leaky gut because their immune system is seeing things it shouldn't be exposed to.

Your immune system has different branches, just like the military.

There is the immunoglobulin E (IgE) branch, which is like the Marines. IgE comes out guns a-blazing with a strong and swift response. An example is if you are allergic to shellfish. As soon as you eat a shrimp, your face swells, you can't breathe, and you're going to the ER. It's obvious, fast, and often life-threatening.

Then, as I mentioned, there is the IgA branch, which is like the Army because it's on the front lines. It's everywhere your body interacts with the outside world–your skin, mouth and GI tract, and respiratory tract. IgA has a frontline defense of guys ready to respond if anyone dares cross the border. Or think of this branch like the bouncer at the door of the club, deciding who's safe to come in and who has to stay out. He'll get into a big fight to keep someone out if he has to. IgA does that in your gut.

Lastly, there is the immunoglobulin G (IgG) branch, which I liken to the Navy. It is stealthy, slow to respond, and often you don't even know what hit you; like a submarine attack that the enemy never knew was there. Just as the submarine keeps moving toward something new, IgG does the same thing. It doesn't have lifelong memory; it often fades away and goes off to attack something else.

The IgG response often attacks foods inappropriately during times of active leaky gut. The difficulty with this attack is that it isn't obvious. The response is usually delayed by 48-72 hours and isn't life-threatening. It often presents as an annoying symptom like headaches, eczema, brain fog, depression, fatigue, anal itching, or stubborn weight loss resistance.

The bigger issue?

These immune responses turn on the "inflammatory cascade," which leads to systemic inflammation. The result? Weight loss resistance or weight regain. So, every time you eat a food that your IgG system has created antibodies against, it's like adding fuel to a fire and restarts that inflammatory process. That is why most elimination diets are at least four weeks long because that's how long it takes to calm down your IgG immune system and stop that attack.

The answer to stopping all this inflammation? Heal your gut. My FTF program is going to help you do that!

If you have read up to this point, then you are definitely ready to accept the challenge that God has set forth. I have no doubt that you can make it through the 40-Day Awakening program and emerge as a better version of yourself; one who has connected with the Trinity on a deeper level than you thought possible!

Are you feeling a stirring in your body? Is your mind racing with thoughts of possibilities or regret? Is your soul nudging you to make a change?

A sense of urgency

> "Do you know what the number one prerequisite for change is? A sense of urgency." –John Kotter, international speaker and New York Times-bestselling author

Since practicing functional medicine, I have felt a sense of urgency to bring you the truth as I now know it!

Why?

Because every day another woman tells me her story of how conventional medicine is failing her, how she is so confused about nutrition, and she no longer trusts her body.

We must stop this!

I have no doubt you are reading this book and it's put a pit in your stomach. You have that guttural feeling because you have experienced what I'm talking about.

You have gone to your doctor because you don't feel like the amazing, vibrant woman you know God created you to be, and you've been dismissed and told that nothing is wrong with you, or worse yet, you've been given pills or had surgeries only to feel the same or worse.

I invite you to consider doing my 40-Day program. I will walk you through it step by step, telling you exactly what to focus on, what to avoid, and more importantly, how to rely on God and His Word for your strength through it all.

Surely goodness and mercy shall follow me all the days of my life, and I shall dwell in the house of the Lord forever.

–Psalm 23:6

Chapter 6

Your Innate Intelligence

God created our bodies with incredible innate intelligence. He gave our bodies the ability to be metabolically flexible, so we could walk 40 days in the desert and survive on our stored fat, or hunt, gather, feast, and disperse the fuel sources to the necessary places in our body. Unfortunately, we have tried to destroy that innate intelligence by living on the SAD diet.

Many of us want to lose weight, but we are stuck in sugar-burning mode; meaning if we don't eat every few hours we feel "hangry," jittery, irritable, and are unable to think straight.

Sugar is toxic to the brain. When we live on cereal, muffins, bagels, donuts, alcohol, sports drinks, juices, and granola bars, we struggle to think and are constantly distracted by thoughts of obtaining more sugar. We grab a bag of chips or crackers to curb the addiction. We drink pop (soda) or have a piece of candy to suck on. All day, every day we ride the sugar roller coaster and wonder why we feel miserable, can't lose weight, and feel weak, frustrated, and hopeless.

Healthy fats are the more stable fuel source. When we burn fat for fuel, we don't have a sharp rise in blood sugar, we don't trigger a big insulin response, we get more calories per gram, and we feel satiated longer. Pairing healthy fats with protein helps keep our ghrelin hormone low. Ghrelin is the appetite-stimulating hormone made from the stomach. Starting our day with fat and protein sets us up for success. We don't make ghrelin as quickly and we don't ride the sugar rollercoaster—we ride in a Bentley on cruise control.

My popular herbal blend Metabo Lift helps relieve hunger pains and is great at getting over those hunger pains when you are transitioning from being a sugar-burner to becoming a fat-burning machine. Consider using Metabo Lift on your journey! You can find it on www.gutsygyn.com or you can scan the QR code at the end of the book.

This feels so much better. Our brain likes ketones (the by-product of fat burning) for fuel, as opposed to excess sugar, which you now know creates inflammation and is the leading driver of chronic diseases like obesity, diabetes, heart disease, and dementia.[29,30,31]

Once I understood the concept of being a sugar-burner or a fat-burner and changed my diet, my health significantly

[29] Nguyen TT, Ta QTH, Nguyen TKO, Nguyen TTD, Giau VV. Type 3 Diabetes and Its Role Implications in Alzheimer's Disease. Int J Mol Sci. 2020 Apr 30;21(9):3165. doi: 10.3390/ijms21093165. PMID: 32365816; PMCID: PMC7246646.

[30] Singh DD, Shati AA, Alfaifi MY, Elbehairi SEI, Han I, Choi EH, Yadav DK. Development of Dementia in Type 2 Diabetes Patients: Mechanisms of Insulin Resistance and Antidiabetic Drug Development. Cells. 2022 Nov 25;11(23):3767. doi: 10.3390/cells11233767. PMID: 36497027; PMCID: PMC9738282.

[31] Zhang YR, Xu W, Zhang W, Wang HF, Ou YN, Qu Y, Shen XN, Chen SD, Wu KM, Zhao QH, Zhang HN, Sun L, Dong Q, Tan L, Feng L, Zhang C, Evangelou E, Smith AD, Yu JT. Modifiable risk factors for incident dementia and cognitive impairment: An umbrella review of evidence. J Affect Disord. 2022 Oct 1;314:160-167. doi: 10.1016/j.jad.2022.07.008. Epub 2022 Jul 19. PMID: 35863541.

changed. I broke up with sugar, declared war against gluten because of my autoimmune condition, and embraced the idea that I wanted to honor God by caring for the body He gave me. I wanted to nourish it instead of treating it like a trash can.

Once you start eating enough healthy fats and protein, you will also be able to break up with sugar and get off the roller coaster. You will be able to give up the snacks and eat only three times per day. You will eat sugar the way God made it—as complex carbohydrates, which are sugars paired with fiber to stabilize your blood sugar.[32] This is the difference between eating an orange and drinking orange juice. If the fiber is removed, then your blood sugar spikes. Fiber prevents our blood sugar from going too high from natural sugars. That's why I suggest to only eat carbs with fiber.

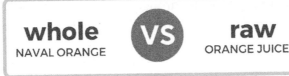

whole	VS	raw
NAVAL ORANGE		ORANGE JUICE

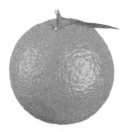
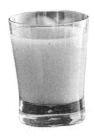

calories	60 kcal	calories	130 kcal
fiber	3 g	fiber	0.5 g
carbs	12 g	carbs	25 g
vitamin c	83 mg	vitamin c	39.5 mg

32 Riccardi G, Rivellese AA, Giacco R. Role of glycemic index and glycemic load in the healthy state, in prediabetes, and in diabetes. Am J Clin Nutr. 2008 Jan;87(1):269S-274S. doi: 10.1093/ajcn/87.1.269S. PMID: 18175767.

Let's visit some basic ideas:

Sugar-burner: Utilizing sugar and carbohydrates as our main source of energy to produce ATP or energy. This is done through frequent eating of sugar and carbs. If we don't use all that energy right away, it gets converted into stored fat throughout our body.

Fat-burner: Using fat (either our stored fat or fat we are eating), instead of relying on sugar, as our main source of energy production. This is how fat loss happens.

The ketogenic diet: Eating fat as our main source of energy to produce ATP or energy-using ketones.

Metabolic-flexibility: Having a body healthy enough to go back and forth between sugar-burning and fat-burning. Being able to utilize the fuel coming in through food, but also easily tapping into our stored fat during times of fasting to burn our own fat as fuel. This is where the magic lives!

Mind your metabolism

Our metabolism is controlled by our thyroid, the master gland. Our thyroid is constantly surveying the landscape of our entire body. It is receiving input from all the other systems (especially the adrenals, nervous system, and gut like I explained earlier) and deciding where to send resources. Our body is either in a state of survival or a state of thrival; it can't be in both.

Thrival describes the state of a healthy metabolism–having metabolic-flexibility, having a creative, open mind, and having a faith-based heart. I believe thrival requires an ongoing relationship with God, listening to the Holy Spirit who is trying to work through us, accepting the unconditional forgiveness that Christ's life has given us, and taking back control of our body, choices, thoughts, feelings, behaviors, and subsequently, our outcomes.

God expects us to take responsibility for the current state of our lives and the future that He is trying to give us. Here's the thing, we have free will. We can choose to not live a God-centered life. He still loves us and has plans for us, but until we want that for ourselves, it won't be activated.

God has an amazing future laid out for you. Will you live into that amazing, fulfilling future or will you settle for a lesser version than what God has planned for your life?

If our body doesn't think there are enough resources coming in to thrive then it will slow down our metabolism. This is seen during times of chronic stress, like caring for a sick parent, working a third shift job, hating your job because you are being bullied every day, or overworking your body training for a marathon. This is also seen when we have gut infections, chronic viruses, too many heavy metals getting into our body, toxic mold exposure, or active autoimmune conditions.

Most commonly, this is seen with the SAD diet and eating too often because this high-sugar, high-calorie, nutrient-depleted diet tells the body there are no nourishing resources so we should eat more and hold onto what we're taking in. The body says, "Don't release any weight, she's starving us to death."

Please look at this picture that I've created. It represents the basis of which I learned from The Cleveland Clinic Institute for Functional Medicine. Our body holds onto our weight by down-regulating our thyroid production. Our thyroid makes thyroxine hormone (better known as T4, the inactive form of thyroid hormone) in response to signals from the brain and other organs. Our body must then convert T4 into triiodothyronine (better known as T3, the active form of thyroid hormone). T3 acts like the gas pedal in our body. It increases (speeds up) our metabolism, increases gut peristalsis so we digest our food and move our bowels, it increases brain activity so we can think and perform functions, it grows our hair and nails, and it tells our ovaries whether it's safe to ovulate or not. It affects all your systems, as well as bone health, heart health, and muscle health.

But, remember our amazing innate intelligence that God put into our bodies? T4 can also be made into rT3 (reverse T3), which is like putting our foot on the brake. It decreases (slows down) our metabolism, slows our bowels, slows our brain function, prevents ovulation, and slows just about every other function in the body. For example, that is why our skin becomes dry and cracked and our hair falls out when we have hypothyroidism.

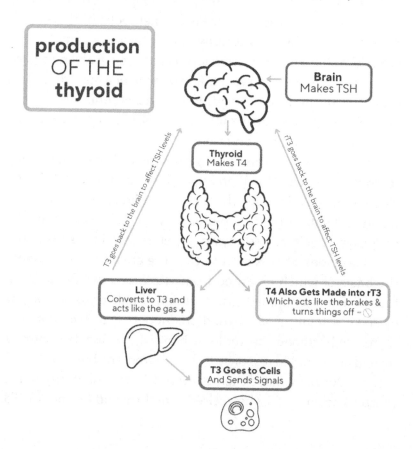

Our body isn't doing this because it doesn't know how to work anymore. **Our body does not betray us.**

It's doing this as a protective mechanism to maintain homeostasis and divert resources to the areas they are most needed. If you have diabetes, yeast overgrowth in your gut, a tooth infection, or aren't getting restorative sleep, then your body isn't going to burn fat for fuel and lose weight. It's going to slow down that process and focus on what needs to be healed.

So many of us are frustrated that we can't lose weight or we are gaining weight and we act like our body is betraying us. On the contrary, **we are betraying our body by not listening to it.**

Weight gain and weight loss resistance is a symptom—a warning sign from our body—trying to tell us that something needs to be dealt with. But instead of honoring our body and thanking it for the information, we shame it, hate it, and continue to expose it to the things that are destroying it.

Please stop beating yourself up.

We have been programmed by our broken society to focus on the wrong things. From this day forward, I want you to give yourself grace and realize that you were doing what you knew. Now, you know better. Like Maya Angelou said, "When you know better, you do better."

Stop doing this...	Start doing this...
Eating the bread/rolls at a restaurant	Tell the waitress not to bring it to the table
Drinking ice water with your meals	Drink hot water with lemon
Taking the elevator	Take the stairs
Criticizing parts of your body you don't like	Thank God for the body parts you do like

Waiting until the right time to change	Start a new habit today
Thinking a doctor is going to heal you	Believe that you have the tools to heal yourself
Giving up because you aren't perfect	BEGIN AGAIN - every day!

After caring for thousands of women, I have come to realize that over 70% of healing comes from simply making different daily choices. When I am evaluating a patient and determining the root cause(s) of their issues, I order functional tests to evaluate the gut microbiome, digestive function, a 24-hour adrenal cortisol pattern, hormone metabolites, food sensitivity testing, and hair testing for heavy metal burden and mineral imbalances. There are always imbalances, dysfunction, and disease processes to reverse. I have never done a functional test on a patient that didn't show something. This means there is work to be done.

Your body is always trying to maintain a state of homeostasis despite everything it endures. Often that homeostasis turns into pure survival and no thrival. The key point is that those dysfunctional processes are because of poor daily choices over a long period of time, which means that returning to thrival (healthy function or healing) requires NEW and different repeated daily choices over a long period of time.

Consistency creates change.

Consistency can create bad change, like a decline in your health. Consistently eating bagels for breakfast, chips for lunch, and drinking soda, sweet tea, or energy drinks creates insulin resistance that can develop into diabetes. On the contrary, consistently eating healthy fats and protein for your first meal creates a strong, satisfied body that isn't controlled by sugar cravings. Consistently sitting all day causes weight gain, muscle loss, poor posture, decreased lung capacity, and stagnant lymph and blood flow, all which can lead to blood clots, infections, falls, injuries, and cancer. On the contrary, consistently moving your body with purpose everyday creates a strong body you can depend on.

What side of consistency do you want to be on?

Accepting two truths

The first truth: You are a holy Trinity. Just as God, Jesus, and the Holy Spirit work together for your healing and salvation, so are you a body, mind, and spirit working together for your healing and salvation.

This is a mantra I say in my head. I would encourage you to say it, too, or create your own because it's a powerful way to start changing what your mind is thinking and believing.

I am more than my physical body. My body was given to me by God to do great things during my time on this earth. My soul should control my mind and hence my body. I have control over my choices every moment of every day because God is always with me, giving me the strength I need to choose right.

Too often we are letting our bodies control our minds and spirits. We need to get in tune and listen to our bodies, but we also need to discern what is worth paying attention to and what is not. Asking the Holy Spirit to live within you and walk along with you every step of the way will make this much easier.

The second truth: You have the choice between living in the light (God) or in the darkness (enemy). That is the free will given to us in the garden of Eden.

As soon as we make the right choice, our soul must fight the darkness, which is always telling our mind to talk our body out of the plan. The enemy will use our mind to try to talk us out of the healthy choice we made. Our soul will tell us to wake up at

5am and go to the gym. When 5am comes, the enemy will tell us we're too tired, that we didn't sleep enough, or that it doesn't matter anyway because we aren't capable of change. We must ignore that chatter. We must fulfill our promise to mature our soul by doing what it wants us to do to grow into the butterfly we are meant to be. The following scripture tells us we need to use our free will and choose. It is a powerful reminder that we need to choose Jesus every morning when we wake up.

God is light; in him there is no darkness at all. If we claim to have fellowship with him yet walk in the darkness, we lie and do not live by the truth. But if we walk in the light, as he is in the light, we have fellowship with one another, and the blood of Jesus, his Son, purifies us from all sin." –1 John 1:5-7

Do you not know that your bodies are temples of the Holy Spirit, who is in you, whom you have received from God? You are not your own; you were bought at a price. Therefore, honor God with your bodies.

–1 Corinthians 6:19-20

Chapter 7

Frankenfoods Versus Faith Foods

Whether your goal is to lose weight, overcome some major health challenges, or just get closer to God, this chapter is a must. We have to get back to eating the foods God created for our bodies to thrive. If you focus on all the incredible food He provides, the SAD diet should fall to the wayside, but just in case, here's some basic guidelines for success.

I recommend avoiding all alcohol, fast food, pop/soda, grains (especially gluten), cow's milk products, inflammatory oils, and some higher carbohydrate beans, legumes, fruits, and vegetables for at least six weeks (the length of the 40-Day Awakening program) to stop the inflammation happening within your body.

Remember how I said it takes four weeks to stop the production of an IgG response by your immune system? If you continually avoid something for at least six weeks, that allows your immune system ample time to calm down so your gut can start to heal. This will also force you to eat foods you don't normally eat and because your microbiome loves change and diversity, this will help you reestablish a healthy microbiome.

Most people do well reintroducing the higher-carb fruits and vegetables after the 40 days without weight regain or blood sugar issues if they are consistently keeping their inflammation down by continuing the healthy lifestyle you are about to embark upon. Everyone is unique and has different preferences and requirements for their nutrition. The point is to focus on faith foods that God made and that man has not genetically modified or changed to the point that your body doesn't recognize it.

Once you do my FTF program, your body will be better able to discern between things serving it and harming it.

The truth is, when we feel bad it's very hard to discern what makes us feel any different; we just feel bad or worse in the form of being tired, in pain, sluggish, and bloated. Once we remove all the inflammation and are functioning like a well-oiled machine, it's more obvious when we ingest something that makes us feel bad. I've experienced this firsthand and hear it every day from my patients. Once you go through my program, it will be obvious if eating dairy or beans or grains makes you feel bad. You will no longer tolerate living a less-than-satisfying life and it will be much easier to avoid your trigger foods. Please trust the process.

Foods to avoid for maximum healing: white sugar, corn syrup, high-fructose corn syrup, wheat and gluten, GMO grains, GMO corn, GMO soy, commercialized dairy/beef/chicken/turkey/pork that have been raised on GMO grain feed, commercially caged eggs, trans fats, margarine, vegetable oil, canola oil, sunflower oil, soybean oil, corn oil, safflower oil, beans, legumes, and alcohol.

Focus on nourishment

For decades we were taught to simply count calories to manage our weight. Everyone from doctors to personal trainers had us believing that if we burn more calories than we consume that we would create a calorie deficit and that would in turn cause weight loss. "Eat less, exercise more" has been the kiss of death for millions of people, further driving them into metabolic dysfunction. My friend and mentor, JJ Virgin, does an amazing job of explaining why this doesn't work. She explains in *The Virgin Diet* that, "Our body is a chemistry experiment, not a bank account."

She helps us understand this concept that while calories represent a unit of energy, the source of those calories and the nutritional composition of the foods can have very different effects on our body, including hunger signals, hormone production, metabolism, and overall health. These are the concepts that I have been showing you throughout the previous chapters. By now you should understand that calories aren't just calories. In other words, 300 calories of bone broth doesn't have the same effect on your body as 300 calories of cake because these different calories are providing the body with completely different information and creating an entirely different response from the body's systems.

Did you hear that? Food is information. What you eat determines what your body does.

This understanding of food being information has led to the newest weight loss tactic, counting macros instead of calories. "Macros" stands for macronutrients. As I alluded to earlier, there are three categories of nutrients we eat the most that are our energy sources: protein, carbohydrates, and fats. Protein gives us amino acids, carbohydrates (carbs) give us sugar like glucose, and fats give us fatty acids. Paying attention to how many of these three macronutrients you ingest each day can help shift what information you are relaying to your body and change what you are trying to get your body to do. This can be helpful if you are trying to shift your metabolism, hormone response, hunger cues, inflammation response, and health of your gut microbiome. The specific ratios you need can vary based on factors like age, gender, activity level, and individual goals.

The FTF program is based on macro counting and was created for women north of 40 years, who are living a mostly sedentary, typical American life, who eat some processed foods, who are looking to lose weight, to decrease the inflammation in her body, and reverse any disease processes that have started. If you are younger and looking to preserve fertility or you are highly phys-ically active, then you would want more carbohydrates during this program. I discuss and teach these nuances in the online version, so please check it out if you'd like more guidance.

I would like to acknowledge that some of us have a history of food restriction, such as an eating disorder, or have person-alities that can go down a slippery slope when doing things like counting calories, macros, or weighing ourselves regularly. I would encourage you to take some time to reflect on your relation-ship with food. Figure out whether you are an emotional eater, if you have negative feelings toward food, if you are afraid of food because you don't understand how it affects you physically and mentally, or whether you are just too busy to think about food and see it as a nuisance.

Now ask God to help you overcome your issues. Ask Him out loud and write it down on paper. Get clear on the obstacle or fear or whatever it is that you've identified. Then, ask for a new under-standing, a new way of handling things, a new response to old triggers, or whatever your soul is crying for. Finally, I would then encourage you to continue reading to understand the basics of counting macros and how the different macros nourish your body in different ways for different reasons, because the more you understand why and how your body responds to what you put in it, the more control you will have in how you feel and whether you will age with health or with disease.

Ultimately, I want you to get to the point where you are eating intuitively and not having to count macros. This requires understanding how your body reacts to different foods, breaking up with sugar, killing the cravings, and getting into harmony with your body. I am going to teach you how to let your soul run the show, instead of your human body's desires driving your choices. Gaining freedom from food will open up a whole new, beautiful way of living for you!

Macros: protein, carbohydrates, and fats

As I explained earlier, carbohydrates are the body's primary source of energy. When you consume carbohydrates, your body breaks them down into glucose, which can be used immediately for energy or stored in the muscles and liver as glycogen for later use. Glucose derived from carbohydrates is the quickest fuel source for your brain and central nervous system. As we age, especially after menopause, our brains tend to function more clearly using ketones from fatty acids.

Proteins are essential for building and repairing tissues. Proteins are composed of many amino acids connected. These get broken down into their individual amino acids and then are used to synthesize new proteins, enzymes, hormones, antibodies, immune-related molecules, and organs like muscle and skin.

Fats are a key component of cell membranes and are required for the transport of nutrients and energy in and out of the cells. Fats are essential for hormone production. And lastly, fats can be turned into ketones for long-term energy and brain food. This is the basis of the ketogenic diet. You are going to learn how to regain your metabolic flexibility, meaning you can go from burning carbs for fuel to burning fats for fuel. Metabolic flexibility is the key to successful fasting.

ATP: Adenosine triphosphate, also known as ATP, is a molecule that carries energy within cells. It is the main energy currency of the cell. All living things use ATP. In addition to being used as an energy source, it is also used in signal transduction pathways for cell communication and is incorporated into DNA during DNA synthesis.[33]

Some important biochemistry: The oxidation of one gram of fat produces more than twice as much ATP (energy) as the oxidation of one gram of carbohydrate. That means eating fat gives us more energy to get through our day. Fat is essential to repair our cells because it is the backbone of our cell membranes (a phospholipid bilayer). Also, all our steroid hormones (like estrogen, progesterone, testosterone, DHEA, cortisol, and aldosterone) are made from cholesterol.

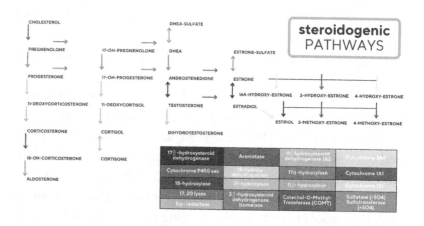

---

33   Dunn J, Grider MH. Physiology, Adenosine Triphosphate. [Updated 2023 Feb 13]. In: StatPearls [Internet]. Treasure Island (FL): StatPearls Publishing; 2023 Jan

Did you know? Our nerves have a protective myelin sheath around them that allows electrical impulses to transmit quickly and efficiently along the nerve cells. (It works like the coating around a wire). The myelin is made of fat and protein. If the body chronically doesn't have enough fat or protein, these coverings can be damaged and our nerves won't function properly. The disease MS is an example of myelin destruction.

Eat these faith foods

Healthy carbs: lettuces, arugula, spinach, Swiss chard, radicchio, zucchini, mushrooms, cucumbers, broccoli, cauliflower, Brussel sprouts, cabbage, asparagus, alfalfa sprouts, squash, radishes, tomatoes, red, yellow, green and orange peppers, celery, blueberries, strawberries, blackberries, raspberries, watermelon, beets

Healthy proteins: grass-fed beef, free-range eggs, wild-caught fish (anchovy, bass, codfish, haddock, halibut, mackerel, perch, snapper, salmon, sole, swordfish, trout, tuna, walleye pike), wild-caught seafood (prawns, crab, shrimp, lobster, mussels, oysters, scallops, clams, squid), free-range chicken and turkey, organ meats, venison, duck, bison, lamb, veal, organic soy, organic tofu, organic tempeh, organic miso, goat's or sheep's milk and cheese

Healthy fats: almonds, avocados, Brazil nuts, cashews, coconut oil, chestnuts, chia seeds, flaxseed, ghee, grass-fed butter, hazelnuts, hemp, macadamia nuts, olives, MCT oil, olive oil, pecans, pistachios, walnuts

Healthy herbs & miscellaneous: basil, black pepper, black tea, cilantro, cinnamon, cloves, cocoa, coffee, dill, fennel seed, ginger, ginseng, green tea, herbal teas, horseradish, licorice, mustard, nutmeg, oregano, paprika, parsley, peppermint, rosemary, sage, tarragon, thyme, turmeric, vanilla bean

Gut-healing foods: fermented foods like sauerkraut, goat's milk kefir, organic miso, low-sugar organic kombucha, fermented pickles, bitters, herbs like ginger, turmeric, fennel, aloe, prebiotic fibers from avocados, garlic, leeks, onions, shallots, scallions, flaxseeds, jicama, chickpeas, lentils

Many people who are used to eating the SAD diet cannot tolerate large amounts of these fermented and prebiotic foods initially. If eating them causes you to have gas and bloating, then you need to nourish your microbiome and add these foods back into your diet slowly. Start with a few bites per day, then one serving per day to see how you tolerate it. As your beneficial bacteria, aka good microbiome, grows and gets reestablished, you should be able to increase these foods.

Preferred sweeteners: Agave, applesauce, chicory, dates, coconut sugar, raw honey, maple syrup, and black-strap molasses. You really shouldn't need to add many sweeteners to your foods because they are whole foods that will be flavored from the natural fats, herbs, and seasonings.

No matter how you are feeling about changing up what you are eating, whether you are excited and all-in or are hesitant and scared to death, please read the next chapter! God has amazing shifts waiting for you for your journey of life. I'm going to lay out the other pieces of my 40-Day Awakening program, so you can start to see how powerful our God is and how you can find so much strength in Him if you just lean in and say yes to yourself.

Let's face it, you not only deserve to do this for yourself, but you also need to do this for yourself. The many wonderful people who you love and care about rely on you. They need you to be healthy and happy. You have lived a selfless life and put others before yourself so many times. You have sacrificed your health and peace of mind for others, just as Jesus has taught, but Jesus also taught us to forgive and nourish ourselves. Jesus spent time alone connecting with God and renewing His mind. Jesus also walked miles every single day and chose clean, nourishing food for His body. We need to use and treat our body the way God intended.

Okay, now that you understand why you are choosing this awakening, it's time to jump in!

Therefore I tell you, whatever you ask for in prayer, believe that you have received it, and it will be yours. –Mark 11:24

Chapter 8

Future Gazing with God

I am going to outline exactly what you need to do to awaken your soul, awaken your physical healing, nourish your relationship with God, and build unstoppable faith with an unstoppable body.

There are four phases, each 10 days long: Sunrise, Transition, Freedom, and Enlightenment. You will focus on five areas throughout all four phases: Your food, daily movement, sleep, cultivating self-love, and strengthening your relationship with the Trinity. Believing in God is one thing, but having an active on-going relationship with the Holy Spirit, and truly living into the forgiveness of Christ is another level. This process is going to bring you there.

There are the seven steps you are going to use as you move through my FTF program. It's called the FAITH IT™ approach:

Fast for focus
Ask for guidance
Ink it for clarity
Thank God for His unconditional love
Hear His plan and desire for you
Initiate action
Trust that He is making a way for your victory

When we fast, we ask God to guide us with every decision, we write down our struggles and desires, we give Him thanks that He is always working in our favor, and trust His timing and decisions. Only then can we hear what He is calling us to do. We initiate action, glorifying Him in our daily actions, and trust that He is protecting us and making our crooked paths straight.

I have seen an endless number of people stuck in self-judgment, self-deprecation, self-loathing, and even self-hatred. I'm here to tell you that you cannot heal a body you hate. And you can't change a life that you don't accept responsibility for.

Know that God created you on purpose, for a purpose. You may have strayed, but He expects that; we are humanly flawed. He wants us to require His presence in our lives. God wants us to need Him.

As soon as I understood that and said, "Lord, I have abused, neglected, and taken my healthy body for granted. Please show me how to love it, nurture it, and heal it," that is when the magic began to happen.

New people, books, podcasts, resources, and opportunities started showing up in my life. When you wake up and ask God for what you need, He will deliver. Are you ready to wake up and pay attention?

You obviously asked Him for something to bring this book to you now. What is it you are searching for? What are you trying to heal?

Maybe you're saying, "I don't even know."

The best way to figure out what you need is to get out of your head; get out of the circle of repeating thoughts that drive confusion and unrest. When we think about things we often get stuck on the problem and aren't able to see the solution because our mind is like a record player; it plays the same thing over and over. It hasn't heard the solution yet, so it can't play it. The way to hear the solution is to write down the problem and ask God to show you the solution. Then—here's the most important part—have faith. Have complete faith that your Father will provide the solution for you, His beloved child.

Seeing yourself through God's eyes

So how do you get out of your head? You write it down.

Open your FTF Journal and fill out the left column of the first chart; this is all the stuff that is bothering you about your body and your life. (If you don't have the journal, then get a piece of paper and draw a vertical line down the center.) The left side is for the words that describe what you do not like about yourself and your situation. Be 100% honest and real. This is for you and God alone. Let the judgment go. God already knows what you're going to write, so don't be ashamed—own it.

Now you are going to fill out the right side of the column. Write down words that describe the complete opposite of what you wrote on the left. Describe exactly how you want to look, feel, be, and live. It's time to get crystal clear about the woman you want to become. See her in your mind's eye. Gaze into the future through God's eyes. How does your beloved creator and Holy Father see you?

What bothers you about your body and life?	How do you want to look, feel, be, and live?
Overweight	Lean, toned, and strong
Tired	Energized
Sad and lonely	Joyful, surrounded by loved ones
Frustrated and overwhelmed	Organized, productive, and calm
Broke, living paycheck to paycheck	Wealthy, blessed, giving back

The more clarity you create, the easier it will be for your brain to lead your body to the right choices. This will become clearer as we progress. I do this mental exercise once a month to make sure I am future gazing through God's eyes so I can become the woman He wants me to be.

Faith it 'til you make it!

Now write a letter to God. This is laid out nicely in the FTF Journal, but again, you can use a piece of paper. I wrote an example below. You can be as specific as you want or need to be. The most important part is to just simply write. Make the pen move. If you don't have a thought, write, "Dear God, please give me a thought. Please help me write what I need from you." Just keep writing until you feel satisfied that your soul is heard. If you need to start with all the things that are bothering you, then write them down, but then start writing down what you want instead. If you are overweight, write, "Thank you God for giving me a body capable of transforming. I know I can lose 10 pounds, 30 pounds, or 100 pounds."

Make sense? You got this!

Dear God,

Thank you for showing me this new path of possibilities. Thank you for giving me the motivation to read Fast to Faith. Thank you for making me brave enough to write this letter. God, I want to be healthy. I want to be the best version of myself that you envisioned for me when you created me. I want to truly love myself again like I did when I was little, before the sins of this world tainted my pure heart. Holy Spirit, please come into my physical body so I may feel you guiding me every step of the way. When I stray, please talk to me. Let me hear my intuition, which is You, Holy Spirit, and guide me back to where I need to be.

Amen

You can use this guide to fill in the blanks for the words I have underlined:

Dear God,

I envision my body as <u>healthy</u>, <u>strong</u>, <u>beautiful</u>, and able to do anything I want it to, not limited or disappointing to me. I envision a future where my <u>joints don't hurt after I exercise</u>, where my <u>stomach feels content and satisfied when I eat</u>, and where I feel <u>energized and alive when I fast</u>.

I know you long to give me all the blessings of this earth including <u>health</u>, <u>vitality</u>, <u>abundance</u>, <u>joy</u>, and <u>connection</u>. I now believe I am worthy. I am now ready to receive these blessings. You sent Your only Son, Jesus Christ, to live amongst us and pay the ultimate price for our human sins so we may know Your grace, Your forgiveness, and Your blessings.

Lord, I am not worthy to receive You, but only say the word and I shall be healed.

Thank You, Jesus, for <u>paving the way for me</u> to enjoy an amazing life of abundance. I accept Your ultimate sacrifice and gift of forgiveness.

Thank you, Holy Spirit, for coming into my heart and <u>helping me hear and see the truth</u>. I am worthy because I am a child of God. Period. End of story. It is time for me to live that truth. It is time to treat my body in a way that honors You, dear Lord.

I am capable.

I am enough.

I am fully equipped.

Amen.

Reboot your hard drive for metamorphosis

The answers all lie within you because God is within you. The ability—the tools you need—all lie within you because God is within you.

Even when we don't acknowledge Him or we cast Him aside, God is always there, working in the background. He coded us. He is like the hard drive in a computer—we can't run without Him. Remember learning how to use a computer? You figured out how to send an email, search on the internet, or save photos. You realized it had many capabilities that you had never utilized. You didn't know how it was all happening internally, but you knew that if you pressed the "Enter" key that the email would send. God is like the hard drive in our computer, providing our coding and our information.

If you turn on your faith computer, He will go to work and do incredible things you didn't even know were possible. Just because you don't know about your abilities, doesn't mean they aren't there. Call on God to help you activate them!

God created us to change. Think about all the wonderful attributes of a child who has been raised in a safe and loving environment. I picture a sweet child running around, laughing, singing, climbing trees, and jumping into a lake without a care in the world, calling out for you to come join them because they are so happy and present in the moment. They are curious, fearless, joyful, brave, imaginative, playful, inviting, inclusive, accepting, inquisitive, and full of boundless energy, flexibility, and health. *That* is the life I crave, so I ask God to make me like His child again. Pray with me.

Dear God,

Release me from all the fears instilled in me, release me from all the hurts I've endured, and forgive me for all the wrongs I've done. I accept Your unconditional love, forgiveness, and guidance.

Amen.

Think of yourself like a caterpillar. Caterpillars are doing fine, living life, eating leaves, and walking around without any real purpose, but they have huge potential inside of them. They eventually get removed from their environment and are wrapped in a protective cocoon. They are broken down into a pile of goo, nourished, and built into something entirely new. Once God has done His job, an incredibly beautiful butterfly emerges to fly away and live an entirely new life. That old caterpillar could only see the ground in front of her and now she soars the skies, seeing new horizons and possibilities and reaching new heights.

Be a butterfly.

God is offering you a metamorphosis. He's waiting for you to ask and receive the transformation. I believe that is why we are here physically on this earth.

Now that you're realizing what your body, mind, and soul are capable of, I implore you to complete my Fast to Faith: A 40-Day Awakening. It will not only transform your physical health, but also your spiritual health.

> "Trust the process. Lean in and do all the things. You will be amazed at the outcome and won't want it to end." –Mandy M., a member of the Fast to Faith Sisterhood

"Preparation is the compass that guides you through the darkest moments and leads you to the light."

–Unknown author

Chapter 9

Prepare for Success

It's time to clean out your pantry and get rid of tempting Frankenfoods. This is essential for your success, especially if you need to break up with sugar or salty snacks. You need to remove the temptation. If you are anything like me, I can't have certain things in the house because I can't eat just one gluten-free Oreo. I have to eat an entire row, so I just don't tempt myself and don't keep them in the house. If that stuff doesn't bother you, then cheers! Either way, let's focus on keeping your fridge stocked with fresh healthy options of God's faith foods!

Go shopping

Buy faith foods such as: leafy greens, cruciferous vegetables, squash, sweet potatoes, grass-fed beef, free-range eggs, wild-caught fish and seafood, free-range chicken and turkey, organ meats, nuts, seeds, avocados, olives, olive oil, coconut oil, MCT oil, basil, cilantro, and parsley.

There is a shopping list and recipes for every single day to simplify the program when you join the online program using the QR code at the end of this chapter.

Drink enough filtered water

Aim to drink at least half your body weight in ounces of filtered water every day. If you weigh 180 pounds, then you should drink at least 90 ounces of filtered water each day. We need to filter the water to remove the toxins, xenoestrogens, and pathogens, but filtering can also remove important minerals and electrolytes, so I will explain how to replace those.

According to The U.S. National Academies of Sciences, Engineering, and Medicine, they determined that an adequate daily fluid intake is 11.5 cups a day for women and 15.5 cups a day for men. These totals account for the fact that we get water from other sources, too, such as tea, coffee, milk, juice, fruits, vegetables, and alcoholic beverages. That means if you are decreasing your consumption of juice or alcohol or giving up milk, then you might need more water intake. This is a conservative recommendation. Please realize that we are composed of water, and therefore it's required in all parts of our body to function.

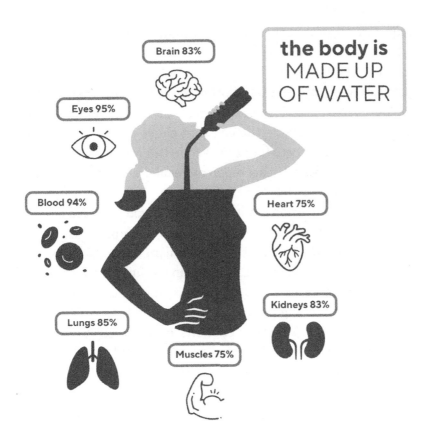

Just as important are the electrolytes that help water maintain its osmolality, meaning the water flows to the areas of the body you want it to and not to other areas. When you have an imbalance, then you develop conditions like edema, elevated blood pressure, and in worse case scenarios, congestive heart failure.

Frankenfoods are high in sodium and chloride and low in potassium and magnesium. This creates an electrolyte imbalance, which shifts where the water in your body goes. This is how eating a bag of potato chips every day contributes to hypertension (chronically elevated blood pressure) and lower extremity edema (leg swelling). The excess sodium, inflammatory oils, and high carbohydrate content cause inflammation and an electro-lyte imbalance that causes water to leave the blood and seep into the other tissues. The inflamed arteries have to use more pressure to pump the blood, thereby increasing their cardiac output. When arteries get inflamed, there are chemical reactions happening inside the cell that cause damage to the cell and affect its ability to function. When this happens repeatedly, then cholesterol and other repair molecules arrive to start repair work, like I talked about in Chapter 4.

For the science nerds out there like me, you know it's actually way more complex. In addition to the Renin-Angiotensin-Aldo-sterone System (RAAS), the mechanism in the kidneys that controls our blood pressure, new research is finding that the cells that line the arteries (endothelial cells) have multiple chemical processes happening according to how many electrolyte mole-cules are around. All those reactions, in various combinations, contribute to increased arterial tone and total vascular resis-tance (TPR) and, hence, elevated blood pressure.[34]

Add electrolytes

My favorite electrolyte replacement to drink every day during this 40-day transformation is Electrolyte Synergy (check it out in my free resources) because it has the right balance of elec-trolytes needed when adopting fasting as a way of life.

---

[34] Blaustein MP, Leenen FH, Chen L, Golovina VA, Hamlyn JM, Pallone TL, Van Huysse JW, Zhang J, Wier WG. How NaCl raises blood pressure: a new paradigm for the pathogenesis of salt-dependent hypertension. Am J Physiol Heart Circ Physiol. 2012 Mar 1;302(5):H1031-49. doi: 10.1152/ajpheart.00899.2011. Epub 2011 Nov 4. PMID: 22058154; PMCID: PMC3311458.

Replace trace minerals, vitamins, and support healing

My favorite supplement is Energy Lift from my Gutsy Gyn collection. Not only does it provide you with the multivitamins and methylated B vitamins you need to metabolize your hormones, but it also has the trace minerals you lack when drinking filtered water. It also contains N-acetyl-cysteine (NAC), which is an important ingredient to make glutathione, your body's major antioxidant that goes around your body and heals damaged cells. Energy Lift also contains other antioxidants like resveratrol, EGCG, ALA, and broccoli seed extract. It also contains inositol, which helps with blood sugar and insulin regulation.

In order to support your body's return to health during this 40-day program, I have put together a FTF Fasting Accelerator Collection that I highly recommend everyone add to their plan. These supplements are so helpful, especially if you are struggling with weight loss resistance, low energy, trouble concentrating, or waking during the night.

Supplementation is often necessary to support your body's detox pathways and replace necessary vitamins and minerals that are most likely deficient from eating a SAD diet. Even if you have been eating a healthy diet composed of clean proteins, vegetables, and fats, these foods may now be deficient in the necessary levels of vitamins and minerals meant to help us thrive because we have overused and depleted our soil. One study states that up to 80% of magnesium is lost during food processing.[35] Another study points out that chronic magnesium deficiency is associated with hypertension, fatal heart attack,

---

[35] Cazzola R, Della Porta M, Manoni M, Iotti S, Pinotti L, Maier JA. Going to the roots of reduced magnesium dietary intake: A tradeoff between climate changes and sources. Heliyon. 2020 Nov 3;6(11):e05390. doi: 10.1016/j.heliyon.2020. e05390. PMID: 33204877; PMCID: PMC7649274.

and stroke.[36,37] This is because magnesium is required for over 300 processes in the body. Vitamin and mineral deficiencies are one of the most common root causes of chronic disease.

Also, as I explained previously, the world we live in is constantly bombarding us with toxins. Our bodies have to expend a lot of energy (using vitamins and minerals) to detoxify from things such as fragrances in our beauty and cleaning products, plastics that package our foods and seep into our drinks, and we need to actively support our body's ability to remove these toxins every day. Because of this reason, basic supplementation is often the missing link for women trying to overcome their health challenges. For me personally, it was a game changer when I was trying to overcome my adrenal fatigue, hormone imbalance, and chronic gut issues.

This realization led to me researching the supplement industry. I found that all supplements are not created equally. It's imperative to take high-quality supplements that are third-party tested for purity, efficacy, and potency. If you take something from the local drug store or look for the best sale online, then you run the risk of taking things that have impurities like heavy metals, gluten fillers, and inconsistent doses of what you are trying to take. These additives will sabotage your progress. This is precisely why I created the Gutsy Gyn supplement line using a top leading manufacturer in the wellness space to ensure these standards are being met and that I can stand behind what I recommend. And remember, even though I am a physician, I am not your physician. I always recommend that you

---

[36] Roberta Cazzola, Matteo Della Porta, Michele Manoni, Stefano Iotti, Luciano Pinotti, Jeanette A. Maier, "Going to the roots of reduced magnesium dietary intake: A tradeoff between climate changes and sources. Heliyon, Volume 6, Issue 11, 2020, e05390, ISSN 2405-8440, DOI: 10.1016/j.heliyon.2020.e05390.

[37] Wanli Guo, Hussain Nazim, Zongsuo Liang, Dongfeng Yang, "Magnesium deficiency in plants: An urgent problem," The Crop Journal, Volume 4, Issue 2, 2016, Pages 83-91, ISSN 2214-5141, DOI: 10.1016/j.cj.2015.11.003.

consult with yours before starting any new supplements, diets, or exercise regimens.

Here is how to use what's in the FTF Fasting Accelerator Collection:

Energy Lift: Take two capsules in the morning and two capsules around noon for foundational cellular function and healing.

Mag Lift: Take two or three capsules before bed and again during the day if desired for sleep support, blood pressure support, proper hormone metabolism, or help relieving headaches or restless legs, among other benefits.

Metabo Lift: Take two capsules 30 minutes before your first meal for appetite control and weight loss support.

Inflamma Tame: Use one scoop daily to help decrease inflammation, regulate bowels, and get enough protein.

Electrolyte Synergy: Pour one scoop in 10-16oz of water in the morning to replace necessary electrolytes depleted during fasting. May repeat during the day as needed.

Additional support, if needed:

Gluco Tame: Take three capsules with dinner every evening to support blood sugar and insulin regulation. This provides excellent support for people with elevated blood sugar, insulin resistance, prediabetes, and diabetes. This supplement contains berberine, which has been shown to lower blood sugar levels and possibly slow the development of diabetes.[38] If you are taking any diabetes medications, please consult your physician before adding this supplement. You most likely just need closer monitoring, such as wearing a continuous glucose monitor (CGM). If you are interested in getting a CGM without a prescription please check out my resources page www.fasttofaith.com/resources or scan the QR code at the end of this chapter.

Biome Lift: Take one capsule twice a day for bowel regulation. This blend of beneficial bacteria is a great probiotic for women struggling with weight loss.

Omega Lift: Take one capsule one to two times a day for added omega-3 fatty acids DHA and EPA for powerful anti-inflammation support.

Digestive Lift: Take two capsules at the beginning of each meal. This is helpful if you struggle with bloating immediately after eating, feel like food sits in your stomach for too long, have cramping with diarrhea soon after eating, see undigested food in your stool, have anal itching, or brittle nails. Please speak with your physician before taking this supplement if you have a history of stomach ulcers.

Join the FTF Online Program and Sisterhood: Consider joining the live online FTF program, which walks you through the program day by day, has educational videos of me explaining the changes happening in your body as you go from being a sugar-burner to a fat-burner, how this impacts your health and hormones, and how to troubleshoot issues when transitioning.

---

[38] Wang Y, Liu H, Zheng M, Yang Y, Ren H, Kong Y, Wang S, Wang J, Jiang Y, Yang J, Shan C. Berberine Slows the Progression of Prediabetes to Diabetes in Zucker Diabetic Fatty Rats by Enhancing Intestinal Secretion of Glucagon-Like Peptide-2 and Improving the Gut Microbiota. Front Endocrinol (Lausanne). 2021 May 7;12:609134. doi: 10.3389/fendo.2021.609134. PMID: 34025574; PMCID: PMC8138858.

We also have a certified functional nutritionist and health coach holding your hand and guiding you to success. The online version has so many helpful resources that I wasn't able to put into this book. We also have an ongoing Sisterhood of support that you can join, which fuels your continued progress after the 40-day program is complete!

Please check out my resources page www.fasttofaith.com/resources or scan the QR code below.

"I believe that the greatest gift you can give your family and the world is a healthy you."

– Joyce Meyer

Chapter 10

Honor God In All Aspects

To truly reconnect your body, mind, and soul, you must become mindful of how you are using your body throughout the day and how you are nourishing or neglecting it. Not only does this account for the food you are putting into your body, what toxins you are exposing it to, but also how you are moving and sleeping. Fasting should also be about avoiding all the things that are harming you, keeping you stuck both physically and mentally, and blocking your relationship with God.

Movement

If you are already exercising or moving your body with purpose every day, continue doing that. If you don't do anything scheduled or consistent, then walk for at least 15 minutes after every meal. If your schedule won't allow that, then make time for one longer walk at some point during the day. If you sincerely can't fit that into your day at all, then you need to take a hard look at your life and your priorities. God wants you to care for the body He lent you for your time on this earth.

One of the best gifts my mom ever gave to me? She said, "I take care of my body now so that hopefully I don't have to burden you with the job of taking care of it later."

She has seen too many people her age struggling with their physical health because they abused their bodies and she sees how their grown children have had to sacrifice their time and energy and physical health to care for them.

Not only do you honor God when you care for your body, but you also honor those you love—your partner, your parents, your children, your friends, and your coworkers—because when you are suffering the consequences of poor daily choices, those are the people who have to set aside their dreams, goals, and plans to help care for you.

Please don't misunderstand me. I would be honored to care for my mother if and when she needs me to. But too often older adults need help sooner and more than they should because years of poor daily choices and habits manifested in chronic ailments, conditions, injuries, and limitations.

We are burdening ourselves and our loved ones unnecessarily. Don't you want to prevent that if you can for as long as you can?

Important note: Every single time you choose something different than your "record player of a mind" knows and understands, it will try to stop you. Your mind will tell you every reason why you shouldn't do it and too often our mind wins the argument.

When I wanted to be the person who wakes up every morning before my family to exercise and spend time with myself this is what happened. I would have every intention of going. I would set my alarm clock and plan to wake up, but when the alarm went off, I allowed my mind to talk me out of it.

But it feels so warm here in my bed and it's so cold outside. I didn't sleep long enough and I can get another hour right now... I'm sore from yesterday, so I should take a break.

I would listen and believe my mind and not work out. Then later I would feel regret, shame, and defeat for not being stronger. I finally realized that I had to make important things non-negotiable.

If we want something, we have to clearly define it, determine our plan, and follow through with it. I realized that I didn't have to listen to my "record player of a mind" and the excuses that kept me stuck. I realized that our mind is afraid of change. Remember, it's a computer program, and it wants to run its program. It will talk us out of things. That is how we become comfortable in our discomfort.

Once I realized this, I decided I could rely on The Holy Spirit and quick decision making to get me through. I finally started going to the gym at 6am and it felt amazing. I felt great physically, but more importantly, I was no longer feeling defeated, mentally weak, or regretful.

Here's what I do: I start the night before and when I am laying there ready to fall asleep, I pray:

Dear God, please give me amazing, healing, restorative sleep and wake me up at 6am with boundless energy and excitement to go work out and love on my body. Thank you, God, for putting me to sleep and waking me up healthier.

Not only do I ask God for help, but I also tell my cells the plan and how to behave because, remember, your cells are listening to your thoughts and producing chemicals accordingly. As soon as the alarm clock wakes me up, I say, "Thank you God. I GET TO exercise."

As I am saying it, I get up. No lingering so there is no opportunity for my mind to talk me out of it. As I am walking to the bathroom, getting dressed, drinking water, brushing my teeth, I am thanking God for my body.

"Thank you, God, for my strong legs, thank you for my beautiful arms, thank you that gravity is no longer winning, thank you for the ability to move so easily, thank you for the energy that moving my body gives me for the rest of the day."

Let me be totally honest here: There are some days when I don't feel that way. I am in pain, I am tired, or I don't have the energy. This moment is the greatest opportunity for you to grow and love the person God created you to be!

When you choose the comfort of familiarity and staying stuck, your brain replays all the lies in your head, "You are weak, you can't get well, you will never lose weight..." and you lose hope, you lose faith, and you no longer believe in or see the possibilities.

When you choose the new, hard, uncomfortable thing, something miraculous happens. Your hope and faith grow, your belief in yourself grows, and your mind starts to see possibilities—possibilities of a brighter, happier, healthier, more abundant future. I want that for you. God wants that for you. I know you want that for yourself.

I always encourage activity in the morning, but I encourage you to choose something you can actually enjoy (sometimes after getting used to it for a bit) like yoga, lifting weights, Pilates, doing a HIIT class, Chi Gong, or walking. If you struggle with the idea of big changes, I recommend waking up 15-20 minutes earlier than you currently are and do it every day. You can slowly add 5-10 minutes until you are eventually waking up an hour earlier. On the other hand, if you are an all-or-none type of person, then I recommend that you just wake up an hour earlier and do it every day. Say your complete sentence as you get out of bed, "Thank you, God. I GET TO exercise."

Thank Him for getting you up and to your workout area and celebrate the little wins. Another idea is to do this with someone you like and hold each other accountable. You are more apt to stick with a healthy habit like morning exercise if you're doing it with a community. That is why my online FTF program has been transformative for many women.

Rely on God for the strength you don't realize you have, and you will be amazed at what you are capable of!

> "I love being in a community of women all working toward the same purpose - both the physical journey and the spiritual journey." –Andrea M., member of the Fast to Faith Sisterhood

Your morning

Getting good, restorative sleep actually starts in the morning. Your body is equipped with an internal clock that runs your sleep-wake cycle, your energy production, your hormone production and utilization, your detoxification pathways, your digestive system, and your healing processes. It's important to live in sync with this clock as much as possible. This is called your circadian rhythm.

In the morning, you should go outside and immediately get sunlight into your eyes. When the sunlight hits your retinas, it stimulates the cortisol awakening response (CAR). This surge of cortisol is like your body's own cup of coffee. It gets you going for the day. If you can't function without one or two cups of coffee, that is a clear sign that your CAR has become stunted or dysfunctional. You must intervene before this gets any worse! Get outside and get that sun in your eyes. If it's dark in the mornings, like where I live in Michigan for many months, then you can do a bio hack. You can buy a full-spectrum white light and shine it in your direction for the first 10-15 minutes each morning to stimulate the CAR.

This beneficial cortisol spike can also increase your blood sugar in a fasted state. I see this often in my groups when women are tracking their glucose and ketones with a device like a Keto-Mojo or a continuous glucose monitor (CGM). They often complain that their fasting glucose goes up in the morning. This is your body's innate intelligence again. It knows that once you are awake, it requires energy to function. If you don't have enough ketones from burning fat, then it will actually make glucose in your liver and put it into your bloodstream so you have enough fuel to start your day.

Say you start your day out super stressed. You didn't wake up early enough or you didn't plan your morning, so you're running around trying to get ready and you spill your coffee all over you. Now you have to take the extra time to change your clothes and put your other clothes in the wash, but you forgot to empty the washer last night because you were too tired. Now you're really late and feeling even more stressed imagining the looks and attitude you're going to get once you walk into work.

When we are stressed, our cave-woman brain (the amygdala) takes over and can only focus on one thing: fight or flight. That is why we can't think clearly when we are stressed. Our amygdala tells our liver to make glucose and puts it into our bloodstream. The problem is that you don't actually fight or flee, so now your body has all this glucose in the bloodstream and no physical activity to use it on because you're just at your desk stewing over your stressful morning, or your boss' frustrating comments, or your overwhelming schedule for the day. Now your body has to make insulin to help take that glucose out of your bloodstream and find a place to store it as fat.

Yep. Stress can make you fat.

You don't even have to eat a SAD breakfast. You could skip eating all morning and eat a clean lunch and dinner, but if you are living a stressed life, your body is making extra glucose, elevating your blood sugar, requiring too much insulin production and driving insulin resistance, obesity, and diabetes.

Mindfulness

> *"For God did not give us a spirit of timidity, but a spirit of power, of love, and of self-discipline." –2 Timothy 1:7"*

God wants you to be intentional.

Mindfulness is a popular term right now, but it was created by God. He wants you to be mindful of everything you do and why you do it. Becoming mindful will set you up for success. It will make mornings enjoyable and productive as opposed to stressful and exhausting. Mornings are a great time to move your body and use your mind. You have all that fuel and a clear head.

Open your FTF Journal and write down what you are currently doing most mornings–how you feel, what energy you give into the world, and how this affects the rest of your day and the people around you. Answer these questions: How do you feel when you wake? What do you accomplish? How do you affect others around you? What energy are you contributing to the world? How does this impact the rest of your day and their day?

Now write what you *want* your mornings to be like. Be bold. Get creative. Think of your dream life! Answer these questions: How do you *want to* feel when you wake? What do you *hope to* accomplish? How do you *want to* affect others around you? What energy *do you want to* contribute to the world? How *will* this impact the rest of your day and their day?

An excerpt from my actual journal eight years ago:

Dear God,

Please help me be a morning person. I want to wake up with energy, work out, and be strong and sexy. I want to laugh with my kids as they get ready for school. I want to get to the office on time and be present with my patients. I want to have time to sit down and eat a healthy lunch and not be rushed. I want to be done working before dinnertime so I can hang out with my kids, cook them healthy food, and help them with their homework. I want to relax in the evening and enjoy what You have created. I want to ride my bike, go to the beach, and hang out with friends. I want to sleep through the night and not get woken up. Please, dear God, help me be this person and live this life.

Thankfully, yours.

With consistency and faith, I stopped living a stressed-out, sleep-deprived, frustrated, unhealthy life and came to live this life I wrote about and prayed for!

Your evening

In the evening, a big reason we have trouble falling asleep or staying asleep is because we eat too close to bedtime. Our body ends up having to digest food at a time when it's supposed to be "cleaning house" and regenerating. This often causes a drop in blood sugar, which causes us to wake up. We see this with alcohol, especially wine, beer, and other high-sugar alcoholic beverages. At first, the alcohol puts us to sleep, but alcohol gets metabolized into sugar, then the sugar gets taken out of the bloodstream and our sugar level drops. That makes us wake up and often we have to urinate and can't fall back asleep.

If you want to sleep better so your body can start healing and preventing disease, then you need to stop drinking alcohol and snacking after dinner. I promise that getting rid of the snacks and drinks after dinner is going to be the game-changer!

Another key to sleeping well is to stop looking at screens (phones, tablets, computers, and TVs) at least one to two hours before bed. When you expose your eyes to a certain type of light at the wrong time, it resets your internal clock.

Some of us have confused our clocks for so long that they're in a different time zone. I often see patients who don't fall asleep until 2am and get up at 4am or 10am or 2pm. They are all clocks that have been reset because the inputs they've been receiving have been consistently wrong.

If you consistently go to bed too late, your clock will adjust to the new schedule because it's always trying to stay on time, but it doesn't mean your body's functions are going to respond to the new times appropriately. Your body was created to wake with sunrise and sleep with the sunset. That is how your physiology is wired. This resetting of the clock often shows up as cortisol awakening response (CAR) dysfunction, fatigue, weight gain, hormone imbalance, infertility, brain fog, and the development of disease.

As part of my 40-Day Awakening program you must reset your clock. Why? Because your stomach has a clock, too, and the smaller clocks (like your stomach clock) sync up with the master clock.

Okay, now that you understand that God has created us to thrive through fasting, are you ready to choose this awakening?

Here's the truth when it comes to fasting– it's not a question of "If" you should fast, but "When." Now I'm going to teach you how.

Let's go!

"Your conviction and your convenience don't live on the same block."

— Lisa Nichols, six-time bestselling author and world renowned motivational speaker

Part 2

Start Your 40-Day Awakening

*T*he Fast to Faith: 40-Day Awakening program is meant to be interactive with God, and ideally, with other women because doing something in a sisterhood magnifies our power and our conviction, and keeps fueling our faith fire so our motivation doesn't dwindle when our willpower runs out. Please check out the online version if you would like to be part of the Fast to Faith Sisterhood of women, led by me, who are going through struggles just like yours. Many have already figured out how to fuel their faith back to healing, health, and harmony.

This program is designed for you to be fed by the living, nourishing Word of God all throughout the day.

You will fast your body while feeding your soul. As I explained earlier, the term fasting can refer to time-restricted feeding (TRF), which means only eating within a certain short window of time, or it can refer to longer times of abstaining from food, such as three to five days. This program is going to ease you into fasting because you must first regain your metabolic flexibility to allow your body to easily get into ketosis and thrive from fasting.

God directed me to use the ancient practice of Lectio Divina to help you meditate on a new scripture each day. This will give you the guidance and power to handle the food choices and lifestyle changes you are about to do. Each day is laid out step-by-step in the online program and in the interactive FTF Journal with room for you to journal and complete the mental exercises.

You have three options for following this program:

1. Follow the basics as laid out in this book.

2. Get the accompanying FTF Journal as a physical resource to read and journal along with the daily Lectio Divina scriptures.

3. Join the online program and get the full, interactive experience of me holding your hand, walking you through each day of scripture meditations, joining our weekly faith building, teaching, and Q&A support Zoom calls, interacting with the other women in the Sisterhood, and getting full access to the amazing recipes and extra resources that can't fit into this book. EVERY WOMAN should be in this online program. God created us to be in community!

The FTF journal and online program can be found at www. fasttofaith.com/resources or by scanning the QR code at the end of the book.

What is Lectio Divina?

Lectio Divina is an ancient method of scripture meditation. It's a simple practice that asks us to let go of our own agenda and ask God to speak to us. This method activates the living, nourishing Word of the Bible for you in your life at this current moment. His Word is alive and active and therefore can speak into your current circumstances.

Please don't try to study the scripture as an observer; instead read it as though God is writing it specifically to you at this moment in your life. What is He saying to you? What message does He want you to hear on this day? What areas of your life do you need to feed? What areas are malnourished, struggling, or dying?

The method of Lectio Divina follows four steps:

Ingest (lectio): Read the passage out loud once through and see what words get your attention.

Digest (meditatio): Read it a second and third time and be curious. When you are reading (or listening with the online FTF program), see what words or phrases stand out to you, see what catches your attention.

Nourish (contemplatio): Ask God, "What are you trying to tell me?" Then write any answer or thoughts that come to your mind.

Grow (oratio): Thank God for His Word, wisdom, guidance, and nourishment. Think about this as many times throughout the day as you can remember to.

Every day for 40 days you are going to do Lectio Divina with the given scripture, along with the food plan I provide. The online version of this program has short three- to five-minute videos that guide you through each Lectio Divina exercise every day.

"For I know the plans I have for you," declares the Lord, "plans to prosper you and not to harm you, plans to give you hope and a future."

–Jeremiah 29:11

Chapter 11

Begin with Sunrise
- Days 1-10

I've titled the first 10 days the Sunrise Phase because we are waking up to new possibilities; new possibilities for our health, our lives, and our relationship with God. Remember, He gives us this new possibility every single day, and it is up to us to decide if we want to wake up and follow His path. I guide you to do that with the daily program, which is laid out in the next section.

I remember listening to a sermon by Joel Osteen that resonated with me. He was talking about how the new day technically starts at midnight when it is still dark. This represents the fact that even in your darkest hour, the light of day will shine upon you. Trust that God will bring you out of the darkness. Don't wait for the light to start anew. The new day starts at midnight, so stop giving excuses and stop procrastinating. Start now. Tomorrow is NOT a better day to start, or next Monday, or when you think you'll feel better. That time will never come. You won't feel better until you do something different. Listening to those excuses (the lies recorded) in your mind is what prevents you from being what God wants you to be. Believe you are strong enough and brave enough to change now.

> Change is hard. Staying stuck is hard. Let's choose the hard that ends in joy and living with the promises God has made to us.

There are two key food components to the Sunrise Phase:

1) Becoming a fat-burner
and
2) Breaking up with sugar (giving up the snacks or frequent eating all day long).

Days 1-5:

Focus on eating three meals a day with **the 2/10/20/30 rule:**

- **2** dashes of sea salt on your food
- **10g Carbs** (fiber gets subtracted): leafy greens, cruciferous vegetables, squash, sweet potatoes, or other root vegetables
- **20g Animal protein**: grass-fed beef, free-range eggs, wild-caught fish and seafood, free-range chicken and turkey, or organ meats
- **30g Fat**: nuts, seeds, avocados, olives, olive oil, coconut oil, MCT oil, grass-fed butter, or ghee

Also focus on:

- **Water**: Drink half your body weight in ounces of distilled water per day.
- **Electrolytes**: 1-2 servings per day, as needed

I want you to eat with the 2/10/20/30 rule **three times per day**. This will remind your body how to burn fat for fuel instead of sugar (carbohydrates). You are going to feel full and satisfied. You can play with this a little bit, too. If you would rather eat 30 grams of carbohydrates during one meal and skip the carbs in the other two meals, that's fine. The point is to decrease your carb intake overall. Remember to subtract the fiber from total carbs, because fiber is good and necessary. That means if the total carbohydrates says 10g and fiber is 5g, then you count that as eating 5 grams of carbs.

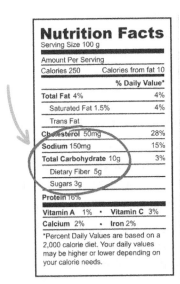

HOW TO FIND
net carbs

EQUATION:
Total Carbohydrates –
Dietary Fiber = Net Carbs

EXAMPLE:
10g - 5g = 5g Net Carbs

Important note: If you had your gallbladder removed or have trouble absorbing fats (you get cramping and/or diarrhea when eating healthy fats) then I recommend you use Digest Lift at the beginning of each meal.

Eating this amount of healthy fat may mentally feel uncomfortable for some people who are stuck in the mindset of calorie restricting or starving oneself to lose weight, or the belief that fat makes us fat. Dr. Mark Hyman did an awesome job of debunking those myths and to show us the truth in his book, *Eat Fat, Get Thin*. If you have those lingering beliefs, I implore you to trust the process. Have faith in yourself, your body, and my FTF program.

Genesis tells us that God gave us incredible food to enjoy from the earth. He provides us with nutrient-dense animals, plants, nuts, seeds, and herbs to thrive. He didn't create all the Frankenfoods in boxes and bags. We did that. God knows best. Trust Him. Eat His faith foods.

> *Then God said, "Let us make man in our image, after our likeness. And let them have dominion over the fish of the sea and over the birds of the heavens and over the livestock and over all the earth and over every creeping thing that creeps on the earth." –Genesis 1:26*

The Word of God is saying that we have been blessed with everything we need. It does not say we are allowed to abuse it, distort it, or dishonor it. Be thankful for the real food you have available and learn to love it the way God desires you to.

My patient, Hannah, did just that. When I first met this 43-year-old woman, she told me that she hadn't had any major traumas in her life and she wasn't overly stressed, but she couldn't understand why she felt seven months pregnant after most meals.

"I exercise and think I'm doing things right, but I'm stuck and can't figure it out," she said.

She joined my FTF program during Lent because, "I felt God telling me that I needed to be more obedient, to fast more often, so I needed the direction and guidance to help me be more obedient in that area."

She had been struggling with cravings, not knowing what or when to eat and she was feeling really discouraged by her lack of results.

By the end of the 40 days, she no longer had cravings, her clothes fit better, and she believed in her body's ability to transform.

"No matter where you are in your health or healing journey, you can adjust the program to meet you where you are and still be blessed," she told me after.

Days 6-10:

Focus on eating three meals a day with the **2/10/20/30 rule:**

- **2** dashes of sea salt
- **10g Carbs** (fiber gets subtracted): leafy greens, cruciferous vegetables, squash, sweet potatoes, or other root vegetables
- **20g Animal protein**: grass-fed beef, free-range eggs, wild-caught fish and seafood, free-range chicken and turkey, or organ meats
- **30g Fat**: nuts, seeds, avocados, olives, olive oil, coconut oil, MCT oil, grass-fed butter, or ghee
- **Water**: Drink half your body weight in ounces of distilled water per day.
- **Electrolytes**: 1-2 servings per day, as needed

AND stop snacking/eating in between those three meals.

Not snacking between meals was really hard for me when I was addicted to sugar and gluten. I downloaded an app on my phone and I started logging everything I ate during the day down to the handful of almonds I grabbed to tide me over. This was eye-opening. I quickly realized I was grabbing things here and there and putting them in my mouth like throwing something in a trash can. Before I started logging my food, I had been eating "breakfast" bars between patients, sharing half a donut with a coworker, filling up my coffee with flavored creamers (sadly, most are full of toxic chemicals) three to four times, sucking on candy after woofing down Taco Bell at lunch or Subway if I was "being healthy," sipping on iced tea or Mountain Dew from 2-4pm, eating a carb-heavy dinner, then having cheese, crackers, chocolate, and wine (when I wasn't on-call) in the evening before bed. It took me logging my food and evaluating the situation as a curious observer to understand how unhealthy my eating habits were. Once I saw this pattern of putting snacks in my mouth throughout the day, I realized just how mindless my eating was.

There was no thought of nourishment and no thought of gratitude or acknowledgement that God was providing all this abundance; I simply came to believe that I should be able to be a glutton whenever I felt like it. If I wanted a candy bar, I should be able to go get one and eat it. I told myself, *What's the big deal? I can afford it... I'm stressed... I'm busy... I deserve it... It's just one candy bar.*

Looking back now, I am ashamed of that entitled way of thinking and more importantly that I was treating my body like a garbage can. I was putting things in my body every day that God did not create to go into my body. My body couldn't function properly when I was fueling it with the wrong stuff.

It's like putting diesel fuel into an unleaded gasoline tank. Putting in diesel will clog the engine. According to an article from capitalone.com, "[The car] will exhibit symptoms like difficulty starting, reduced power, emitting smoke from the exhaust, and potentially causing the catalytic converters to fail."[39]

Our body wants unleaded gasoline (faith foods made by God) but we're fueling it with diesel (Frankenfoods), so our body is exhibiting symptoms like difficulty waking up in the morning, reduced energy, and emitting irregular bowel movements, gas, and belching. These are signs that we're putting the wrong fuel into our bodies. If we don't stop and put in the right fuel, then our catalytic converter (thyroid, heart, brain) will fail.

How to successfully stop snacking

It's important to realize what we are designating as meals. Start writing down or logging into a food app everything that goes into your mouth. An app like Loselt or MyFitnessPal is helpful because it will not only track your food intake, but it will also tell you how many of the three different macros you are ingesting. Remember, macros are carbs, protein, or fats. Changing your ratios is key for feeling full and satisfied when eating, losing weight, helping your body to function properly, heal, and reverse disease processes.

Important note: Ghrelin, our hunger hormone, gets released in a pulsatile fashion. This means the level will rise, make us feel hungry, and will then subside after 15-30 minutes. Yes, it will go away. Ride the hunger wave to the other side by drinking a glass of distilled or electrolyte water, distract yourself with a walk or another form of physical activity, and feel the victory on the other side of not giving into every little temptation your body craves. You are more than your physical body!

---

[39] "What Happens If I Put Diesel Fuel In A Gas Car? Filling up with the wrong type of fuel can be a costly mistake." by Nelson Ireson, December 23, 2022. Capital One Auto Finance (Online Article)

Reframe

"I loved the idea of faith and functional health coming together in one space. This program is a wonderful mind, body, and spirit connection." –Stephanie S., a member of the FTF Sisterhood

When you prepare your food and eat it, I want you to think about all the people who had to work in order for you to enjoy this abundance. Did someone have to pick berries in a field? Did someone have to collect the beans, run them through a mill, package them up, and drive a semi-truck to get them to you? Did someone have to kill an animal, skin, and butcher it? Did someone have to plant the seeds, tend the fields, and harvest them? Did someone dice your onion or cut your fruit at the supermarket so you didn't have to?

You are beyond blessed!

So many people have served you in ways that you take for granted every single day. Start thanking God for these blessings and this abundant life you have. Thank Him while you're making dinner, while you're eating, and while you're cleaning up. We tend to remember a little of this around Thanksgiving or Easter, but we are so blessed all day, every day, and we take it for granted. The following verse is an expression of God's provision and abundance. He provides all our needs, including overflowing our cup. We live a glutenous life and it's time to stop.

> You prepare a table before me
>   in the presence of my enemies.
> You anoint my head with oil;
>   my cup overflows.
> Surely your goodness and love will follow me
>   all the days of my life,
> and I will dwell in the house of the LORD
>   forever. –Psalm 23:5-6

Phase 1: Sunrise Phase (Days 1-10)

Day 1 Lectio Divina

Prayer of Preparation: "Father, help me to be still and enjoy the sunrise of my faith. Just as the sky changes colors, drowns out the darkness, and shines light for us to see each morning, let Your Word enlighten my heart and my mind. Let me clearly see how You want me to nourish my body, my mind, and my spirit."

Ingest: *Then Jesus was led by the Spirit into the wilderness to be tempted by the devil. After fasting 40 days and 40 nights, He was hungry. The tempter came to Him and said, "If you are the Son of God, tell these stones to become bread."*

Jesus answered, "It is written: 'Man shall not live on bread alone, but on every word that comes from the mouth of God.'"

Then the devil took Him to the holy city and had Him stand on the highest point of the temple. "If you are the Son of God," he said, "throw yourself down. For it is written:

> *'He will command his angels concerning you,*
> *and they will lift you up in their hands,*
> *so that you will not strike your foot against a*
> *stone.'*

Jesus answered him, "It is also written: 'Do not put the Lord your God to the test.'"

Again, the devil took Him to a very high mountain and showed Him all the kingdoms of the world and their splendor. "All this I will give you," he said, "if you will bow down and worship me."

Jesus said to him, "Away from me, Satan! For it is written: 'Worship the Lord your God, and serve Him only.'

Then the devil left him, and angels came and attended him.
–Matthew 4:1-11

Digest: Read that again and be curious. See what words or phrases stand out to you, see what catches your attention.

Nourish: Ask God, "What are you trying to tell me?" Then write down what comes to mind. The FTF journal is a great way to keep these writings all together.

Grow: Repeat this prayer, "Thank you God, for giving me your Son, Jesus Christ, so I can know how to live and navigate this complex world. Thank you for showing me the power of faith, conviction, resisting temptations and forgiveness as witnessed by your Son's life. I pray that I come through this 40-Day Awakening program stronger and convicted in my faith, knowing that I am greater than these worldly temptations. Dear Lord, please help me to be more Christ-like and stay rooted in Your Word."

Think about this as many times as you can throughout the day.

Food: Focus on eating at least three meals a day with the 2/10/20/30 rule.

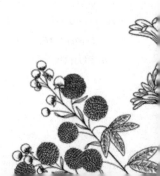

Day 2 Lectio Divina

Prayer of Preparation: "Father, help me to be still and to focus on what You want to say to me. Holy Spirit, open my ears to hear it and open my heart and mind to understand and receive it."

Ingest: *Just as a body, though one, has many parts, but all its many parts form one body, so it is with Christ. For we were all baptized by one Spirit so as to form one body—whether Jews or Gentiles, slave or free—and we were all given the one Spirit to drink.* –1 Corinthians 12:12-13

Digest: Read that again and be curious. See what words or phrases stand out to you, see what catches your attention.

Nourish: Ask God, "What are you trying to tell me?" Then write down what comes to mind.

Grow: Repeat this prayer, "Dear Lord, thank you for reminding me that my body is Your creation and with that comes so much potential for greatness. Thank you for guiding me to this program, so I might focus on how to heal my body and honor You, Father. I pray for strength and conviction in my faith, knowing that I am greater than these worldly temptations. Father, please help me to stay rooted in Your Word."

Think about this as many times as you can throughout the day.

Food: Focus on eating at least three meals a day with the 2/10/20/30 rule.

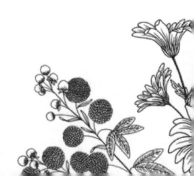

Tabatha Barber, DO, FACOOG, NCMP, IFMCP

Day 3 Lectio Divina

Prayer of Preparation: "Father, help me to be still and to focus on what You want to say to me. Holy Spirit, open my ears to hear it and open my heart and mind to understand and receive it."

Ingest: *"But blessed is the one who trusts in the Lord, whose confidence is in Him. They will be like a tree planted by the water that sends out its roots by the stream. It does not fear when heat comes; its leaves are always green. It has no worries in a year of drought and never fails to bear fruit."* Heal me, Lord, and I will be healed; save me and I will be saved, for you are the one I praise. –Jeremiah 17:7-8, 14

Digest: Read that again and be curious. See what words or phrases stand out to you, see what catches your attention.

Nourish: Ask God, "What are you trying to tell me?" Then write down what comes to mind.

Grow: Repeat this prayer, "Dear Lord, thank you for my beautiful, strong, resilient body. Please teach me to be aware of the negative self-talk happening in my mind; the lies on autoplay that aren't true. Holy Spirit, banish them from my subconscious and replace them with these truths: I am beautiful. I am strong. I am capable of transformation."

Think about this as many times as you can throughout the day.

Food: Focus on eating at least three meals a day with the 2/10/20/30 rule.

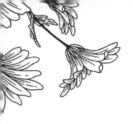

Day 4 Lectio Divina

Prayer of Preparation: "Father, help me to be still and to focus on what You want to say to me. Holy Spirit, open my ears to hear it and open my heart and mind to understand and receive it."

Ingest: *Do not be anxious about anything, but in every situation, by prayer and petition, with thanksgiving, present your requests to God. And the peace of God, which transcends all understanding, will guard your hearts and your minds in Christ Jesus. Finally, brothers and sisters, whatever is true, whatever is noble, whatever is right, whatever is pure, whatever is lovely, whatever is admirable—if anything is excellent or praiseworthy—think about such things. Whatever you have learned or received or heard from me, or seen in me—put it into practice. And the God of peace will be with you. –Philippians 4:6-9*

Digest: Read that again and be curious. See what words or phrases stand out to you, see what catches your attention.

Nourish: Ask God, "What are you trying to tell me?" Then write down what comes to mind.

Grow: Repeat this prayer, "Thank you God, for your unconditional love and never-ending presence. Thank you for the abundant blessings you have given me and continue to give me every day. Holy Spirit, please help me to focus on the body and health that I desire. Help me to make choices all throughout the day to make it happen. I believe in myself because I have the power of the Holy Spirit inside me."

Think about this as many times as you can throughout the day.

Food: Focus on eating at least three meals a day with the 2/10/20/30 rule.

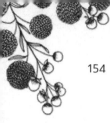

Day 5 Lectio Divina

Prayer of Preparation: "Father, help me to be still and to focus on what You want to say to me. Holy Spirit, open my ears to hear it and open my heart and mind to understand and receive it."

Ingest: *I know what it is to be in need, and I know what it is to have plenty. I have learned the secret of being content in any and every situation, whether well fed or hungry, whether living in plenty or in want. I can do all this through Him who gives me strength. –Philippians 4:12-13*

Digest: Read that again and be curious. See what words or phrases stand out to you, see what catches your attention.

Nourish: Ask God, "What are you trying to tell me?" Then write down what comes to mind.

Grow: Repeat this prayer, "Thank you, Lord, for reminding me that I am strong and capable of anything. In You, I am nourished and complete. Please show me how to nourish my physical body in a way that pleases You, Dear Lord. I am devoted to being the amazing woman You created me to be!"

Think about this as many times as you can throughout the day.

Food: Focus on eating at least three meals a day with the 2/10/20/30 rule.

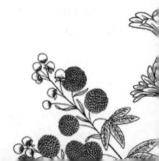

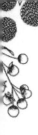

Day 6 Lectio Divina

Prayer of Preparation: "Father, help me to be still and to focus on what You want to say to me. Holy Spirit, open my ears to hear it and open my heart and mind to understand and receive it."

Ingest: *But He gives us more grace. That is why Scripture says: God opposes the proud, but shows favor to the humble.*

Submit yourselves, then, to God. Resist the devil, and he will flee from you. Come near to God and he will come near to you. Humble yourselves before the Lord, and he will lift you up. –James 4:6-8, 10

Digest: Read that again and be curious. See what words or phrases stand out to you, see what catches your attention.

Nourish: Ask God, "What are you trying to tell me?" Then write down what comes to mind.

Grow: Repeat this prayer, "Thank you dear God, for showing me my human shortcomings. Thank you for sending your only Son to pay for my sins, so I may be blessed with Your forgiveness. Please give me the courage to step into the amazing future You have waiting for me; a future of health, joy, beauty, success, and abundance."

Think about this as many times as you can throughout the day.

Food: Focus on eating at least three meals a day with the 2/10/20/30 rule and eliminate snacking between meals.

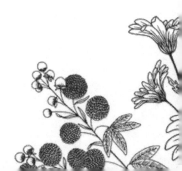

Day 7 Lectio Divina

Prayer of Preparation: "Father, help me to be still and to focus on what You want to say to me. Holy Spirit, open my ears to hear it and open my heart and mind to understand and receive it."

Ingest: *All a person's ways seem pure to them, but motives are weighed by the Lord. Commit to the Lord whatever you do, and he will establish your plans.* –Proverbs 16:2-3

Digest: Read that again and be curious. See what words or phrases stand out to you, see what catches your attention.

Nourish: Ask God, "What are you trying to tell me?" Then write down what comes to mind.

Grow: Repeat this prayer, "Dear God, I have complete faith in your timing and purpose for my life. I know that I am meant for more. Please show me the path, introduce me to the people, and give me the resources to accomplish all the dreams you have placed on my heart, Dear Lord."

Think about this as many times as you can throughout the day.

Food: Focus on eating at least three meals a day with the 2/10/20/30 rule and eliminate snacking between meals.

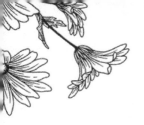

Day 8 Lectio Divina

Prayer of Preparation: "Father, help me to be still and to focus on what You want to say to me. Holy Spirit, open my ears to hear it and open my heart and mind to understand and receive it."

Ingest: *Shortly before dawn Jesus went out to them, walking on the lake. When the disciples saw him walking on the lake, they were terrified. "It's a ghost," they said, and cried out in fear.*

But Jesus immediately said to them, "Take courage! It is I. Don't be afraid."

"Lord, if it's you," Peter replied, "tell me to come to you on the water."

"Come," he said. –Matthew 14:25-29

Digest: Read that again and be curious. See what words or phrases stand out to you, see what catches your attention.

Nourish: Ask God, "What are you trying to tell me?" Then write down what comes to mind.

Grow: Repeat this prayer, "Thank you God, for giving me Your promises in physical flesh. Let me be courageous just as Jesus was when He encountered sin, temptations, and other drama. Dear Lord, give me the strength to believe and the courage to be my authentic self. Holy Spirit, work Your miracles through me."

Think about this as many times as you can throughout the day.

Food: Focus on eating at least three meals a day with the 2/10/20/30 rule and eliminate snacking between meals.

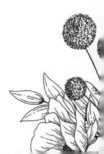

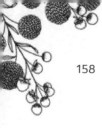

Day 9 Lectio Divina

Prayer of Preparation: "Father, help me to be still and to focus on what You want to say to me. Holy Spirit, open my ears to hear it and open my heart and mind to understand and receive it."

Ingest: *Then your light will break forth like the dawn, and your healing will quickly appear; then your righteousness will go before you, and the glory of the Lord will be your rear guard.* –Isaiah 58:8

Digest: Read that again and be curious. See what words or phrases stand out to you, see what catches your attention.

Nourish: Ask God, "What are you trying to tell me?" Then write down what comes to mind.

Grow: Repeat this prayer, "Thank you God, for believing in me. Thank you for reconnecting my soul and my physical body. Please help me to heal my body and shine my light. Even though I have failed You countless times, You still raise me up and make me whole again. Thank you for giving me a body that heals, that I can honor and nourish all the days of my life."

Think about this as many times as you can throughout the day.

Food: Focus on eating at least three meals a day with the 2/10/20/30 rule and eliminate snacking between meals.

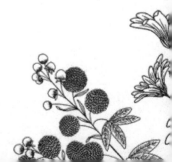

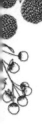

Day 10 Lectio Divina

Prayer of Preparation: "Father, help me to be still and to focus on what You want to say to me. Holy Spirit, open my ears to hear it and open my heart and mind to understand and receive it."

Ingest: *Lord, by such things people live; and my spirit finds life in them too. You restored me to health and let me live. –Isaiah 38:16*

Digest: Read that again and be curious. See what words or phrases stand out to you, see what catches your attention.

Nourish: Ask God, "What are you trying to tell me?" Then write down what comes to mind.

Grow: Repeat this prayer, "Thank you for feeding my soul, which nourishes my physical body. Your love and forgiveness are all I need to survive and thrive, Dear Lord."

Think about this as many times as you can throughout the day.

Food: Focus on eating at least three meals a day with the 2/10/20/30 rule and eliminate snacking between meals.

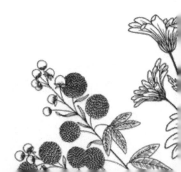

"Through fasting... I have found a perfect health, a new state of existence, a feeling of purity and happiness, something unknown to humans."

–Upton Sinclair

Chapter 12

Move into Transition
Phase 2 - Days 11-20

I want you to realize how incredible your healing ability truly is. Sue is a shining example of this and her story is all too common. Sue is a 57-year-old woman who had a long, complicated medical history. She had spent decades in our broken medical system, seeing different doctors for different complaints, being offered pill after pill and procedure after procedure. She trusted her doctors because that's how she was raised.

"They are in charge and went to school for this, so they must know best," she told herself.

She had her gallbladder removed at age 20 for chronic pain that no one could figure out. She continued to struggle with digestion problems, heavy periods, miscarriages, skin conditions, and weight gain. At 43, she was diagnosed with thyroid cancer and had half of her thyroid removed. Six years later, she had an endometrial ablation for heavy periods, which pushed her into menopause. She was chronically on omeprazole for heartburn, which is a medication to block stomach acid. Unfortunately, that medication was designed to be used in the very short term for symptom control and not to stay on for many months or years. Being on these types of medications too long can cause multiple issues, like bacteria overgrowth in your stomach, parasites not getting killed off that enter your body, improper digestion of food leading to food sensitivities, and vitamin and mineral deficiencies from improper absorption. Sadly, this multi-system dysfunction is an all-too-common scenario, yet no doctor steps back to put all the pieces together and address the underlying reason for why this is all happening.

Sue saw my FTF program and joined in an effort to lose weight, but what she gained was way more than weight loss. She was able to wean off omeprazole because she healed her stomach and esophagus and no longer had the heartburn symptom. She regulated her thyroid and lost 17 pounds during the 40 days. She continued my program as her new lifestyle and is enjoying life again; doing active things like hiking with her boyfriend. She says her friends have commented on how good she looks and how much energy she has.

She recently shared this in the FTF group: "I'm consistently losing half to one pound per week. I hit the lowest weight I've been in 10 years. I am beyond excited how easy these changes have been for me! And, I had an ultrasound on my thyroid a couple weeks ago (I have nodules on my remaining thyroid) and was told it's the best ultrasound the doctor has seen compared to the prior ones. That just blew my mind! To top it off, I just ran a 10k in 1 hour 13 minutes. Your faith will take you farther than you can imagine!"

Whatever you believe is what you will manifest.

Believe you can do this!

Now, for days 11-15, I want you to eat only during an eight-hour window. This is called time-restricted feeding (TRF) in a 16:8 window.

The eight hours starts when you start eating and ends when you stop eating. I recommend that you stop eating at least three hours before going to bed. For many of you, this may be the hardest part. Our evenings are often associated with bad habits, like snacking and drinking alcohol. As I explained earlier, this wreaks havoc on our blood sugar, hormones, sleep cycle, and gut microbiome.

More importantly, these bad habits keep up from having a healthy, flourishing relationship with God. We often feel ashamed of how we waste our time or treat our bodies. We get stuck in a rut. We become complacent and content with our unsatisfying life because change feels more uncomfortable than our current, familiar state of discomfort.

This is your opportunity to see what you're made of!

It's time to shake things up, get uncomfortable, and grow. You are going to grow closer to God, closer to the person God created you to be, and closer to whom your soul longs to be.

Try going for a long walk with your spouse, child, family member, or friend after dinner as a way to reconnect. Or you may want to go alone and use that time to talk to God. Ask the Holy Spirit to be alive and forefront in your life. Here's an example:

> Dear God,
>
> Please continue to help me make better choices. Always point me in the direction of the light and remind me that I am strong enough and brave enough to choose the light. Thank you, Dear God, for believing in me and giving me the tools I need to live into the future I know waits for me. A future full of energy, joy, easy movement,

and a healthy, beautiful body. Thank you for showing me how to release this extra weight, which no longer serves me. Thank you for sending Your only Son to die on the cross, so that I may have forgiveness. Forgiving myself for the gluttony, the mindless living, and the disconnect may be the hardest part, but I know in Jesus Christ I am forgiven, I am made new. There is nothing I can do to earn Your love, You merely give it unconditionally because I have accepted Christ as my savior. Lord, You walk ahead of me and for that I am forever grateful.

Amen.

Isn't Sue's story powerful? Yours can be powerful, too, and I can't wait to hear it!

By the way, congratulations on completing phase one and embarking on the exciting journey of phase two– The Transition Phase. The next 10 days are going to be truly amazing as you continue with your 16:8 eating window and add in the famine-feast carb cycling.

One essential thing to remember during this phase is the importance of distinguishing between carbohydrates and fiber when calculating your daily carb intake. I want you to eat at least 35-40 grams of fiber daily. This distinction is crucial because fiber is necessary for weight management, colon health, having healthy bowel movements (and avoiding constipation), and for the clearance of your used-up hormones.

Please understand that feasting is just as important as fasting!

Day 18 is your famine day, followed by a feast day on day 19. On your feast day, increase your carbohydrate intake to 150-200 grams. This is where many women struggle, and it's an area where conventional diets often fail. We are not small men; our bodies react differently to starvation. We need to remind our bodies that we're not depriving them and we do that with a nourishing feast.

By combining intermittent fasting with carb cycling, you will begin to break through weight loss resistance and low energy. Remember, it's not just about calories. Calories are merely a measure of energy from food. To nourish your body effectively, you need a balance of various nutrients, including B vitamins, magnesium, iron, copper, vitamin C, amino acids, fatty acids, and others. These nutrients are the building blocks that allow your cells to perform their essential functions.

That's why your commitment to this program is crucial. What you feed your body matters, and you'll soon discover just how transformative it can be. You're not just counting calories; you're nourishing your body with the ingredients it needs to thrive.

More importantly, you are nourishing your soul. If you've struggled with self-love, make a promise to yourself and God to work on it. Your body is a gift from God, and honoring it is a way to honor Him. It's okay if you haven't done so in the past. What matters is your commitment to taking better care of your body now. Your choices today are shaping a different future, so celebrate each new decision you make.

The key to lasting change is consistency in your new actions. Embrace discomfort, knowing that God is your support. The online FTF Sisterhood is there to support you as well, just check out the Resources section at the end of the book.

Not only do I believe in you and in your body's incredible ability to transform, but I know it's possible. I would invite you to go beyond believing this for yourself– KNOW it deep down in your soul. Accept it as a fact because that is God's promise to you.

Now live into that promise every day!

Intermittent Fasting: Days 11-17 & 20

- 16:8 Rule: Fast for 16 hours and eat only during an eight-hour window.
- Eat three meals a day by following the 2/10/20/30 rule.

Famine: Day 18

- 22:2 Rule
- You will fast for 22 hours and eat only during a two-hour window. This means you will fast from dinner to dinner, or breakfast to breakfast, or lunch to lunch, whichever works best for your life.

Feast: Day 19

- Eat following the feast rule of 2/50/20/30.
- Enjoy a high dose of healthy carbs during your 16:8 eating window. This 2/50/20/30 rule consists of eating at least 50g of carbs along with your fats and protein, for a total of 150-200g of carbs this day.
- It's important to choose brightly-colored, fibrous foods as your carbs, like sweet potatoes, cabbage, squash, nuts and seeds, quinoa, apples, pears, oranges, grapefruit, grapes, raisins, dates, and figs. Please continue to avoid wheat, oats, corn, rice, and legumes.

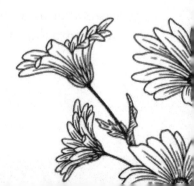

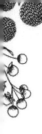

Day 11 Lectio Divina

Prayer of Preparation: "Father, help me to embrace any discomfort as I shift and step into all the incredible changes You have planned for me. Help me to see the unknown as exciting and promising. Holy Spirit, open my ears to hear the promises, open my heart to believe them, and open my mind to receive them."

Ingest: *Everyone ought to examine themselves before they eat of the bread and drink from the cup. For those who eat and drink without discerning the body of Christ, eat and drink judgment on themselves. That is why many among you are weak and sick, and a number of you have fallen asleep. But if we were more discerning with regard to ourselves, we would not come under such judgment. Nevertheless, when we are judged in this way by the Lord, we are being disciplined so that we will not be finally condemned with the world. –1 Corinthians 11:28-32*

Digest: Read it again and be curious. See what words or phrases stand out to you, see what catches your attention.

Nourish: Ask God, "What are you trying to tell me?" Then write down what comes to mind.

Grow: Repeat this prayer, "Dear Lord, thank you for opening my eyes to the fact that I was living as though asleep. Help me to see my shortcomings. Stay ever present in my life. Lord, I need you every hour and every minute of my days."

Think about this as many times as you can throughout the day.

Food: Focus on eating three meals a day with the 2/10/20/30 rule within your eight-hour eating window (the 16:8 rule).

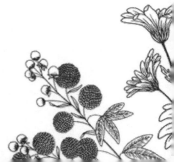

Day 12 Lectio Divina

Prayer of Preparation: "Father, help me to embrace any discomfort as I shift and step into all the incredible changes You have planned for me. Help me to see the unknown as exciting and promising. Holy Spirit, open my ears to hear the promises, open my heart to believe them, and open my mind to receive them."

Ingest: *Therefore, I urge you, brothers and sisters, in view of God's mercy, to offer your bodies as a living sacrifice, holy and pleasing to God—this is your true and proper worship. Do not conform to the pattern of this world, but be transformed by the renewing of your mind. Then you will be able to test and approve what God's will is—his good, pleasing and perfect will. –Romans 12:1-2*

Digest: Read that again and be curious. See what words or phrases stand out to you, see what catches your attention.

Nourish: Ask God, "What are you trying to tell me?" Then write down what comes to mind.

Grow: Repeat this prayer, "Thank you, God, for this amazing body that blesses me every single day and for reminding me to honor and cherish it. Thank you for also making me more than my physical body. As I heal my body, let me also heal my spirit and grow closer to You, Lord."

Think about this as many times as you can throughout the day.

Food: Focus on eating three meals a day with the 2/10/20/30 rule within your eight-hour eating window (the 16:8 rule).

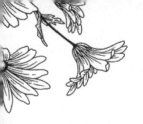

Day 13 Lectio Divina

Prayer of Preparation: "Father, help me to embrace any discomfort as I shift and step into all the incredible changes You have planned for me. Help me to see the unknown as exciting and promising. Holy Spirit, open my ears to hear the promises, open my heart to believe them, and open my mind to receive them."

Ingest: *Consider it pure joy, my brothers and sisters, whenever you face trials of many kinds, because you know that the testing of your faith produces perseverance. Let perseverance finish its work so that you may be mature and complete, not lacking anything. If any of you lacks wisdom, you should ask God, who gives generously to all without finding fault, and it will be given to you. –James 1:2-5*

Digest: Read that again and be curious. See what words or phrases stand out to you, see what catches your attention.

Nourish: Ask God, "What are you trying to tell me?" Then write down what comes to mind.

Grow: Repeat this prayer, "Thank you, God, for the opportunity to be better; to grow and to learn. Through my faithfulness, I know You will bless me with abundance and prosperity."

Think about this as many times as you can throughout the day.

Food: Focus on eating three meals a day with the 2/10/20/30 rule within your eight-hour eating window (the 16:8 rule).

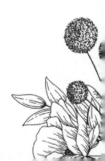

Day 14 Lectio Divina

Prayer of Preparation: "Father, help me to embrace any discomfort as I shift and step into all the incredible changes You have planned for me. Help me to see the unknown as exciting and promising. Holy Spirit, open my ears to hear the promises, open my heart to believe them, and open my mind to receive them."

Ingest: *The Lord will guide you always; he will satisfy your needs in a sun-scorched land and will strengthen your frame. You will be like a well-watered garden, like a spring whose waters never fail.* –Isaiah 58:11

Digest: Read that again and be curious. See what words or phrases stand out to you, see what catches your attention.

Nourish: Ask God, "What are you trying to tell me?" Then write down what comes to mind.

Grow: Repeat this prayer, "Thank you, God, for giving me everything I need for my physical body and my energetic spirit. Thank you for always feeding my body, mind, and soul. Thank you for the abundance of plants and animals that nourish my body and the abundance of Your love that nourishes my soul."

Think about this as many times as you can throughout the day

Food: Focus on eating three meals a day with the 2/10/20/30 rule within your eight-hour eating window (the 16:8 rule).

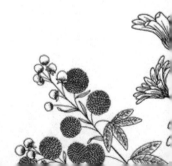

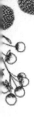

Day 15 Lectio Divina

Prayer of Preparation: "Father, help me to embrace any discomfort as I shift and step into all the incredible changes You have planned for me. Help me to see the unknown as exciting and promising. Holy Spirit, open my ears to hear the promises, open my heart to believe them, and open my mind to receive them."

Ingest: *Never again will they hunger; never again will they thirst. The sun will not beat down on them, nor any scorching heat. For the Lamb at the center of the throne will be their shepherd; he will lead them to springs of living water.' 'And God will wipe away every tear from their eyes. –Revelation 7:16-17*

Digest: Read that again and be curious. See what words or phrases stand out to you, see what catches your attention.

Nourish: Ask God, "What are you trying to tell me?" Then write down what comes to mind.

Grow: Repeat this prayer, "Thank you, God, for leading me to the springs of living water. I am excited to know You more and step into the greatness You have planned for me. Thank you for putting dreams in my heart. Thank you for giving me a body capable of transformation.

Think about this as many times as you can throughout the day.

Food: Focus on eating three meals a day with the 2/10/20/30 rule within your eight-hour eating window (the 16:8 rule).

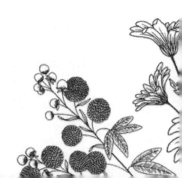

Days 16-20: Add the famine and feast cycle

Over the next few days, you will have one day when you will eat only during a 22:2 eating window (famine day). This means you will fast from dinner to dinner (or lunch to lunch or breakfast to breakfast). Make sure that when you eat you are making good choices and are using the 2/10/20/30 rule.

The next day you will enjoy a high dose of healthy carbs within your 16:8 eating window (feast day). This consists of eating at least 150-200g of carbs along with your fats and protein. It's important to choose brightly-colored, fibrous foods like sweet potatoes, cabbage, squash, nuts and seeds, quinoa, apples, pears, oranges, grapefruit, grapes, raisins, dates, and figs. Please continue to avoid wheat, oats, corn, rice, and legumes.

This was the missing piece for 54-year-old Shelly. She joined the FTF online program and was skeptical because she had been doing intermittent fasting and had plateaued in her weight-loss efforts. She was told by her doctor that her labs were all normal and that she was just getting older.

"Weight gain is a normal part of aging, so get used to it," he told her.

She was also feeling guilty that her weight even mattered to her. "I know it's superficial of me to care about what I look like, but I don't feel good in my body and I'm sick of it."

I, not so tactfully, told her that her doctor was completely wrong. I explained that this myth being perpetuated by the conventional medical community is a flat-out lie. Aging does <u>not</u> cause weight gain. But doctors say that because they don't have any other answer for you thanks to their disease-based model of care. I can say this freely because I was one of them. I know what we're taught in medical school, in residency, and how narrow-minded the medical community is when it comes to weight, health, and nutrition.

Once I found the world of functional medicine, I was quickly reminded of everything I had learned in undergrad with my Bachelors of Physiology degree. I remembered how all the processes in our cells require certain ingredients at certain times and they all work together to produce an outcome. Once we get back to supporting the natural processes God created our bodies to do, we can flourish, reverse disease, and live a balanced life without carrying excess weight.

I explained to Shelly and the group that excess weight is just another symptom. It is your body's way of saying something is off. When Shelly had done the famine-feast cycle and finished Phase 2, she finally started losing weight.

"I believe in my body again. I know it's capable of getting to a healthy weight," she had shared.

Shelly went on to lose another 12 pounds and she has kept it off over the past year. This program will help your body figure that out and finally release that extra weight, too. This program is simply using the tools God gave us and maximizing how to make our bodies run efficiently the way they are supposed to until our last day on this earth.

> "The information about WHY we need to eat healthy, and WHEN and HOW it heals our bodies is invaluable and unlike anything else I have ever experienced! And the daily devotional guide is incredible!" –Sarah V., a member of the FTF Sisterhood

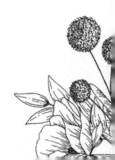

Day 16 Lectio Divina

Prayer of Preparation: "Father, help me to embrace any discomfort as I shift and step into all the incredible changes You have planned for me. Help me to see the unknown as exciting and promising. Holy Spirit, open my ears to hear the promises, open my heart to believe them, and open my mind to receive them."

Ingest: *Blessed are those who hunger and thirst for righteousness, for they will be filled. –Matthew 5:6*

Digest: Read that again and be curious. See what words or phrases stand out to you, see what catches your attention.

Nourish: Ask God, "What are you trying to tell me?" Then write down what comes to mind.

Grow: Repeat this prayer, "Dear Lord, I am so grateful that You brought me on this journey and to this place of gratitude and faith. Father, I want to do right by You. I want to live the life You have planned for me; one of joy, abundance, connection, prosperity, and giving. Thank you for making me Christ's hands to serve."

Think about this as many times as you can throughout the day.

Food: Focus on eating three meals a day with the 2/10/20/30 rule within your eight-hour eating window (the 16:8 rule).

Day 17 Lectio Divina

Prayer of Preparation: "Father, help me to embrace any discomfort as I shift and step into all the incredible changes You have planned for me. Help me to see the unknown as exciting and promising. Holy Spirit, open my ears to hear the promises, open my heart to believe them, and open my mind to receive them."

Ingest: *For this reason, I remind you to fan into flame the gift of God, which is in you through the laying on of my hands.*
For the Spirit God gave us does not make us timid, but gives us power, love, and self-discipline. –2 Timothy 1:6-7

Digest: Read that again and be curious. See what words or phrases stand out to you, see what catches your attention.

Nourish: Ask God, "What are you trying to tell me?" Then write down what comes to mind.

Grow: Repeat this prayer, "Thank you, God, for making me stronger than those temptations. Thank you for showing me how to love my body and care for it. Through You, everything is possible."

Think about this as many times as you can throughout the day.

Food: Focus on eating three meals a day with the 2/10/20/30 rule within your eight-hour eating window (the 16:8 rule).

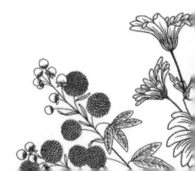

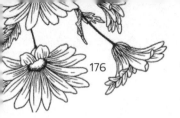

Famine Day: Day 18 Lectio Divina

Prayer of Preparation: "Father, help me to embrace any discomfort as I shift and step into all the incredible changes You have planned for me. Help me to see the unknown as exciting and promising. Holy Spirit, open my ears to hear the promises, open my heart to believe them, and open my mind to receive them."

Ingest: *Therefore, my dear brothers and sisters, stand firm. Let nothing move you. Always give yourselves fully to the work of the Lord, because you know that your labor in the Lord is not in vain. –1 Corinthians 15:58*

Digest: Read that again and be curious. See what words or phrases stand out to you, see what catches your attention.

Nourish: Ask God, "What are you trying to tell me?" Then write down what comes to mind.

Grow: Repeat this prayer, "Thank you, God, for showing me that I am stronger than I once believed. I am powerful and capable because You nourish me. My body is amazing and I am so grateful for it!"

Think about this as many times as you can throughout the day.

Famine Day Food: You will fast for 22 hours and eat only during a two-hour window (the 22:2 rule). This means you will fast from dinner to dinner, or breakfast to breakfast, or lunch to lunch, whichever works best for your life. Make sure when you eat that you are making good choices and using the 2/10/20/30 rule.

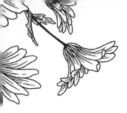

Feast Day: Day 19 Lectio Divina

Prayer of Preparation: "Father, help me to embrace any discomfort as I shift and step into all the incredible changes You have planned for me. Help me to see the unknown as exciting and promising. Holy Spirit, open my ears to hear the promises, open my heart to believe them, and open my mind to receive them."

Ingest: *He said to me: "It is done. I am the Alpha and the Omega, the Beginning and the End. To the thirsty I will give water without cost from the spring of the water of life." –Revelation 21:6*

Digest: Read that again and be curious. See what words or phrases stand out to you, see what catches your attention.

Nourish: Ask God, "What are you trying to tell me?" Then write down what comes to mind.

Grow: Repeat this prayer, "Lord, I need You. You bless me, nourish me, and help me to grow into a woman more incredible than I knew possible. Thank you, Lord, for showing out in my life."

Think about this as many times as you can throughout the day.

Feast Day - Food: Enjoy a high dose of healthy carbs during your 16:8 eating window following the 2/50/20/30 rule. This consists of eating at least 150-200g of carbs along with your fats and protein. It's important to choose brightly-colored, fibrous foods as your carbs, like sweet potatoes, cabbage, squash, nuts and seeds, quinoa, apples, pears, oranges, grapefruit, grapes, raisins, dates, and figs. Please continue to avoid wheat, oats, corn, rice, and legumes.

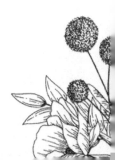

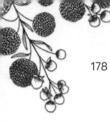

Day 20 Lectio Divina

Prayer of Preparation: "Father, help me to embrace any discomfort as I shift and step into all the incredible changes You have planned for me. Help me to see the unknown as exciting and promising. Holy Spirit, open my ears to hear the promises, open my heart to believe them, and open my mind to receive them."

Ingest: *Then he said to them all: "Whoever wants to be my disciple must deny themselves and take up their cross daily and follow me. For whoever wants to save their life will lose it, but whoever loses their life for me will save it. What good is it for someone to gain the whole world, and yet lose or forfeit their very self?" –Luke 9:23-25*

Digest: Read that again and be curious. See what words or phrases stand out to you, see what catches your attention.

Nourish: Ask God, "What are you trying to tell me?" Then write down what comes to mind.

Grow: Repeat this prayer, "Father, You gave me life at birth and You are giving me life again. I am open and ready to live as the strong, beautiful, talented, and mindful woman You created me to be. I admit I am amazing and capable of anything with the Holy Spirit guiding me."

Think about this as many times as you can throughout the day.

Food: Focus on eating three meals a day with the 2/10/20/30 rule within your eight-hour eating window (the 16:8 rule).

"Fasting is the first principle of medicine; fast and see the strength of the spirit renew itself."

–Rumi

Chapter 13

Kickstart Your Freedom in Phase 3 – Days 21-30

Welcome to Phase 3: The Freedom Phase. It's incredibly liberating and empowering to break free from the constant hold of food. By now, hopefully you've embraced the belief that you can go without eating all the time, and that fasting, even within your 16:8 window, should make you feel good, not deprived.

Fasting isn't about starvation; it's about empowering yourself and trusting in your body's capabilities. God created us to do remarkable things, including periods of fasting. You've already experienced the 22-hour fasting window along with the feast day, which is a crucial part of this journey.

Feast days are just as vital as famine days. They replenish your energy stores and send a signal to your thyroid that you're not starving. As I explained in detail in Chapter 6, your thyroid has the potential to downregulate its functions if it believes you're on the brink of starvation. In this state, your body conserves energy, leaving you feeling tired, fatigued, and constipated. Your hair may become dry and brittle, and your skin may follow suit. These are all signs of a down regulated thyroid. Feast days are designed to prevent this from happening.

So, enjoying carbohydrates and indulging in all the delicious foods that God has created is essential on your feast days. It's not about deprivation or guilt, but nourishing your body in a way that promotes healing, health, and longevity.

Now, let's talk about something really freeing. During Phase 3, we're going to embark on a three-day water fast. Many women are absolutely terrified at the idea of a three-day water fast. As soon as they hear about it, they say things like "There's no way I can do that." Or "I won't be able to function." Or "I might last one day, but not three, no way."

A three-day water fast might sound daunting, but it's about surrendering yourself to God and believing in your body's incredible capacity to go without food. This spiritual and physical transformation is remarkable. Fasting is God's way of allowing your body to heal from the inside out. It's one of the most potent tools for fighting cancer, reversing chronic diseases like diabetes, and stimulating new cell growth. Not only does fasting clear out damaged cells, but it also encourages new cells to regenerate, contributing to your overall health and vitality.

For many people, it is safe to do three-day water fasts or fasting-mimicking diets a few times per year to induce autophagy, manage weight, and improve metabolic health. This approach was made popular by Dr. Jason Fung and Dr. Valtor Longo, who are prominent figures in the field of intermittent fasting and are great resources for understanding all the medical benefits associated with the different types of fasting.

Please note, that while fasting is a great therapeutic tool for healing, I recommend you do these longer fasts under medical supervision and tailor this program to your specific medical needs. Fasting can have potential risks and may not be suitable for everyone, especially those with certain medical conditions. Fasting is not suitable for pregnant or nursing women, children, or the elderly. Even though I am a physician, I am not your physician. Consulting with a healthcare professional before attempting any fasting regimen is crucial to ensure safety and effectiveness.

A three-day water fast is not only a healing journey, it's also an empowering experience that shows you just how capable you are. Women who initially thought they couldn't do it have been surprised by their own strength and self-control. So, approach it with an open mind. Even if you only complete two days, you'll still gain numerous mental, emotional, and physical benefits.

Once you complete the water fast and start reintroducing food, keep in mind that your digestive system has been offline for a few days. Your stomach hasn't been producing the usual digestive enzymes and hydrochloric acid. So, when you begin eating again, opt for foods that are easy to digest. I call this reintroduction soft and slow. Cook your vegetables and meats; enjoy stews, broths, soups, or smoothies. This gentle approach is crucial for your post-fast transition.

I want you to continue to do your daily journaling using Lectio Divina as laid out in the upcoming pages. The companion FTF Journal that is available in the Resources section (at the end of the book) has more detailed pages to guide you during these few days if you are interested. I highly recommend using it or at least writing down how you are feeling, what you are thinking, and what you envision accomplishing through this process. Future-gaze through God's eyes again. This is such a powerful tool to keep you focused.

When you re-ignite your faith and invite Christ back into your life as an active participant, He goes to work. He pours his blessings and favors onto you and you receive blessings that you otherwise wouldn't have.

Stop looking to your own willpower and motivation to do the hard things. God wants you to rely on Him. God wants to use you as an example of His awesomeness, to show the rest of the world how powerful He can be in your life. Please, ask the Holy Spirit to take over for you, direct you, show you the way to health and happiness. God gave you a beautiful, strong, resilient body with incredible innate intelligence. It will heal and transform if you feed it the right ingredients—God's food and God's Word.

I got you. God's got you!

FAITH IT!

Intermittent Fasting: Days 21-24

- 16:8 Rule: Fast for 16 hours and eat only during an eight-hour window.
- Eat three meals a day by following the 2/10/20/30 rule.

Feast: Day 25

- Eat following the feast rule of 2/50/20/30.
- Enjoy a high dose of healthy carbs during your 16:8 eating window. This 2/50/20/30 rule consists of eating at least 50g of carbs along with your fats and protein.
- It's important to choose brightly-colored, fibrous foods as your carbs, like sweet potatoes, cabbage, squash, nuts and seeds, quinoa, apples, pears, oranges, grapefruit, grapes, raisins, dates, and figs. Please continue to avoid wheat, oats, corn, rice, and legumes.

Water Fast: Days 26-28

- These three days will be a longer fast where you completely abstain from food and only drink water, electrolytes, and herbal teas (or follow a minimal calorie fast using recipes I provide in the FTF online program). These days focus on autophagy, physical healing, and spiritual awakening.

Days 29-30: Soft and slow reintroduction of foods

- During these two days, you will focus on eating within your 16:8 window, however, when it comes to what you eat, I suggest you focus on foods that are easy to digest. Some examples include soups, cooked vegetables, broth, and smoothies.

Every woman has a personal reason for wanting to fast their body and feed their faith. What's yours?

Here are a few reasons women have done the FTF program:

- "I wanted to learn more about fasting and combining that with my love of Jesus and my health journey, sounded just like what I needed to be successful and stay on track." –Kristen W.
- "I was drawn to the connection between faith, fasting, health and yes, weight loss!" –Mandy M.
- "I wanted to get better acquainted with scripture."– Cecelia T.
- "I wanted to become more centered in faith." –Sandy S.
- "I was looking for something.... I heard you on a podcast and I just felt the push to join. I was really missing the prayer piece in my life."–Jennifer D.

- "I joined FTF to bring God into my healing and health journey."–Amy S.
- "To greatly improve my health." –Barb V.

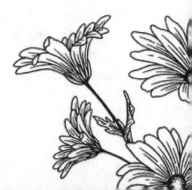

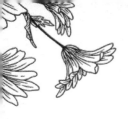

Day 21 Lectio Divina

Prayer of Preparation: "Father, help me to flourish as Your daughter. Continue to guide me with Your living, nourishing Word. Holy Spirit, open my ears to hear the plan, open my eyes to see the path, and open my mind to live into it."

Ingest: *For it is by grace you have been saved, through faith—and this is not from yourselves, it is the gift of God— not by works, so that no one can boast. For we are God's handiwork, created in Christ Jesus to do good works, which God prepared in advance for us to do. –Ephesians 2:8-10*

Digest: Read that again and be curious. See what words or phrases stand out to you, see what catches your attention.

Nourish: Ask God, "What are you trying to tell me?" Then write down what comes to mind.

Grow: Repeat this prayer, "Father, help me to see, feel, and know the power You have given me, so I might conquer my fears and be a shining example of Your miraculous powers. Help me to shut down the lies in my head and only listen to the Holy Spirit."

Think about this as many times as you can throughout the day.

Food: Focus on eating three meals a day with the 2/10/20/30 rule within your eight-hour eating window (the 16:8 rule).

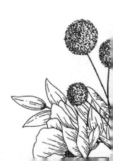

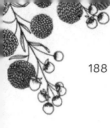

Day 22 Lectio Divina

Prayer of Preparation: "Father, help me to flourish as Your daughter. Continue to guide me with Your living, nourishing Word. Holy Spirit, open my ears to hear the plan, open my eyes to see the path, and open my mind to live into it."

Ingest: *Better a dry crust with peace and quiet than a house full of feasting, with strife. –Proverbs 17:1*

Digest: Read that again and be curious. See what words or phrases stand out to you, see what catches your attention.

Nourish: Ask God, "What are you trying to tell me?" Then write down what comes to mind.

Grow: Repeat this prayer, "Dear Lord, help me to remember what is important as I go through my day. Remind me that earthly pleasures are fine, but what I really crave is the peace only You can give."

Think about this as many times as you can throughout the day.

Food: Focus on eating three meals a day with the 2/10/20/30 rule within your eight-hour eating window (the 16:8 rule).

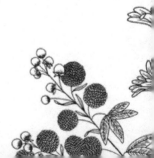

Day 23 Lectio Divina

Prayer of Preparation: "Father, help me to flourish as Your daughter. Continue to guide me with Your living, nourishing Word. Holy Spirit, open my ears to hear the plan, open my eyes to see the path, and open my mind to live into it."

Ingest: *All creatures look to you to give them their food at the proper time. When you give it to them, they gather it up; when you open your hand, they are satisfied with good things.* –Psalm 104:27-28

Digest: Read that again and be curious. See what words or phrases stand out to you, see what catches your attention.

Nourish: Ask God, "What are you trying to tell me?" Then write down what comes to mind.

Grow: Repeat this prayer, "Thank you God, for making me satisfied. I am filled with joy because my soul and body are finally working together. I am living as You created me to live. Please give me more of this every day, Dear Lord."

Think about this as many times as you can throughout the day.

Food: Focus on eating three meals a day with the 2/10/20/30 rule within your eight-hour eating window (the 16:8 rule).

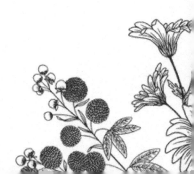

Day 24 Lectio Divina

Prayer of Preparation: "Father, help me to flourish as Your daughter. Continue to guide me with Your living, nourishing Word. Holy Spirit, open my ears to hear the plan, open my eyes to see the path, and open my mind to live into it."

Ingest: *Let love and faithfulness never leave you; bind them around your neck, write them on the tablet of your heart. Then you will win favor and a good name in the sight of God and man. –Proverbs 3:3-4*

Digest: Read that again and be curious. See what words or phrases stand out to you, see what catches your attention.

Nourish: Ask God, "What are you trying to tell me?" Then write down what comes to mind.

Grow: Repeat this prayer, "Thank you, Father, for showing me unconditional love through Your Son, Jesus Christ. Thank you for reminding me daily that I am worthy; that I am enough. I am the daughter of a King."

Think about this as many times as you can throughout the day.

Food: Focus on eating three meals a day with the 2/10/20/30 rule within your eight-hour eating window (the 16:8 rule).

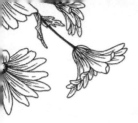

Feast Day: Day 25 Lectio Divina

Prayer of Preparation: "Father, help me to flourish as Your daughter. Continue to guide me with Your living, nourishing Word. Holy Spirit, open my ears to hear the plan, open my eyes to see the path, and open my mind to live into it."

Ingest: *Jesus answered, "I am the way and the truth and the life. No one comes to the Father except through me. If you really know me, you will know my Father as well. From now on, you do know him and have seen him." –John 14:6-7*

Digest: Read that again and be curious. See what words or phrases stand out to you, see what catches your attention.

Nourish: Ask God, "What are you trying to tell me?" Then write down what comes to mind.

Grow: Repeat this prayer, "Thank you, Father, for giving me Jesus. Thank you for expecting more of me and challenging me to act more Christ-like. Thank you for this journey called life. Holy Spirit, please help me to listen and grow closer to my Father every day."

Think about this as many times as you can throughout the day.

Feast Day Food: Enjoy a high dose of healthy carbs during your 16:8 eating window following the 2/50/20/30 rule. This consists of eating at least 150-200g of carbs along with your fats and protein. It's important to choose brightly-colored, fibrous foods as your carbs, like sweet potatoes, cabbage, squash, nuts and seeds, quinoa, apples, pears, oranges, grapefruit, grapes, raisins, dates, and figs. Please continue to avoid wheat, oats, corn, rice, and legumes.

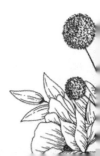

Water Fast: Day 26 Lectio Divina

Prayer of Preparation: "Father, help me to flourish as Your daughter. Continue to guide me with Your living, nourishing Word. Holy Spirit, open my ears to hear the plan, open my eyes to see the path, and open my mind to live into it."

Ingest: *Is this the kind of fast I have chosen, only a day for people to humble themselves? Is it only for bowing one's head like a reed and for lying in sackcloth and ashes? Is that what you call a fast, a day acceptable to the Lord? –Isaiah 58:5*

Digest: Read that again and be curious. See what words or phrases stand out to you, see what catches your attention.

Nourish: Ask God, "What are you trying to tell me?" Then write down what comes to mind.

Grow: Repeat this prayer, "Dear Lord, thank You for the strength to honor You through my sacrifice. Thank you for the incredible ability to change my physical body, to look better and feel better. Lord, thank you for growing my faith and my belief in myself."

Think about this as many times as you can throughout the day.

Water Fast Day 1: You will completely abstain from food and only drink water, electrolytes, and herbal teas (or follow a minimal calorie fast using recipes I provide in the FTF online program).

Journal: Write down what you want to experience today. Make it as amazing as possible. Is it boundless energy? A flat stomach? A lightness to your body? A sense of pride?

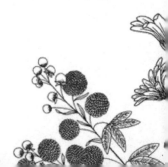

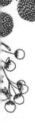

Water Fast: Day 27 Lectio Divina

Prayer of Preparation: "Father, help me to flourish as Your daughter. Continue to guide me with Your living, nourishing Word. Holy Spirit, open my ears to hear the plan, open my eyes to see the path, and open my mind to live into it."

Ingest: *On the last and greatest day of the festival, Jesus stood and said in a loud voice, "Let anyone who is thirsty come to me and drink. Whoever believes in me, as Scripture has said, rivers of living water will flow from within them." –John 7:37-38*

Digest: Read that again and be curious. See what words or phrases stand out to you, see what catches your attention.

Nourish: Ask God, "What are you trying to tell me?" Then write down what comes to mind.

Grow: Repeat this prayer, "Thank you God, for giving me Your Son, Jesus Christ, so I may know Your commitment to me. You believe in me and now I finally believe in me, too. Thank you for showing me what I am capable of. I am strong and unstoppable. My body has innate intelligence to heal. I am connected to the Holy Trinity now and forever."

Think about this as many times as you can throughout the day

Water Fast Day 2: You will completely abstain from food and only drink water, electrolytes, and herbal teas (or follow a minimal calorie fast using recipes I provide in the FTF online program).

Journal: Name all your strengths and accomplishments. What are some things you've done that still surprise you to think about? How did you feel when those things happened?

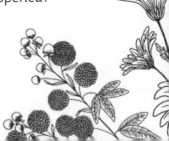

Water Fast: Day 28 Lectio Divina

Prayer of Preparation: "Father, help me to flourish as Your daughter. Continue to guide me with Your living, nourishing Word. Holy Spirit, open my ears to hear the plan, open my eyes to see the path, and open my mind to live into it."

Ingest: *Jesus answered, "Everyone who drinks this water will be thirsty again, but whoever drinks the water I give them will never thirst. Indeed, the water I give them will become in them a spring of water welling up to eternal life." –John 4:13-14*

Digest: Read that again and be curious. See what words or phrases stand out to you, see what catches your attention.

Nourish: Ask God, "What are you trying to tell me?" Then write down what comes to mind.

Grow: Repeat this prayer, "Thank you God, for quenching my body and my soul. Thank you for helping me realize I am greater than my physical desires. I have the power to control how I look and how I feel. Holy Spirit, continue to guide me so I may be the best version of myself that God has envisioned for me."

Think about this as many times as you can throughout the day.

Water Fast Day 3: You will completely abstain from food and only drink water, electrolytes, and herbal teas (or follow a minimal calorie fast using recipes I provide in the FTF online program).

Journal: What will be your biggest challenge today? What are three things you can do to make it easier (i.e., ask for help, meditate, sing, watch something funny, explore nature)?

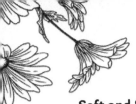

Soft and Slow Reintroduction: Day 29 Lectio Divina

Prayer of Preparation: "Father, help me to flourish as Your daughter. Continue to guide me with Your living, nourishing Word. Holy Spirit, open my ears to hear the plan, open my eyes to see the path, and open my mind to live into it."

Ingest: *"Then you will find your joy in the Lord, and I will cause you to ride in triumph on the heights of the land and to feast on the inheritance of your father Jacob." For the mouth of the Lord has spoken.* –Isaiah 58:14

Digest: Read that again and be curious. See what words or phrases stand out to you, see what catches your attention.

Nourish: Ask God, "What are you trying to tell me?" Then write down what comes to mind.

Grow: Repeat this prayer, "Father, thank you for sending me on this path toward true joy, for it is the fruit of the spirit. Please fill me with joy no matter what comes throughout the day. Help me to stay in peace, knowing that real life and real joy can only be found in You."

Think about this as many times as you can throughout the day.

Soft and Slow Reintroduction Food: Focus on eating within your 16:8 window and choose foods that are easy to digest. Some examples include soups, cooked vegetables, broth, and smoothies. For more examples, join my FTF online program.

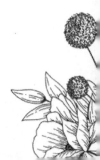

Soft and Slow Reintroduction: Day 30 Lectio Divina

Prayer of Preparation: "Father, help me to flourish as Your daughter. Continue to guide me with Your living, nourishing Word. Holy Spirit, open my ears to hear the plan, open my eyes to see the path, and open my mind to live into it."

Ingest: *A cheerful heart is good medicine, but a crushed spirit dries up the bones. –Proverbs 17:22*

Digest: Read that again and be curious. See what words or phrases stand out to you, see what catches your attention.

Nourish: Ask God, "What are you trying to tell me?" Then write down what comes to mind.

Grow: Repeat this prayer, "Lord, direct my thoughts and actions. Cast out evil spirits and stop the lies playing in my head. Help me to be mindful of how my thoughts direct my feelings and therefore my actions. Keep me ever present to the truth: That I have a choice in everything, every minute of every day. Help me to choose the way of Your Son, my savior, Jesus Christ."

Think about this as many times as you can throughout the day.

Soft and Slow Reintroduction Food: Focus on eating within your 16:8 window and choose foods that are easy to digest. Some examples include soups, cooked vegetables, broth, and smoothies. For more examples, join my FTF online program.

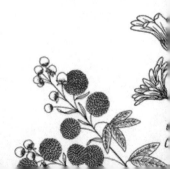

"But those who hope in the LORD will renew their strength.
They will soar on wings like eagles; they will run and not grow weary, they will walk and not be faint."

–Isaiah 40:31

Chapter 14

Become Enlightened - Days 31-40

Welcome to the last phase–Enlightenment Phase! I know you're feeling incredible as you break free from food cravings, shed limiting beliefs, shift negative thoughts, and realize what you are truly capable of when you lean into God for your strength. He wants you to step into your power and realize your potential. He made you for more!

In this final phase, I want you to embrace this as your new way of life. The old you no longer serves you. As God suggests, let go of your past life and enter into a new one with a deep connection to Him and your renewed identity. This is not just about a 40-day plan, it's about creating lasting habits that lead to a sustainable, fulfilling life.

Think about the life you were living before you embarked on this FTF journey. Was that life sustainable? Sometimes we're so caught up in our daily stressors that we don't stop to ask if it's sustainable. I recall a moment when a physical therapist made me ponder this question and it changed my life. Your life should not be breaking you; it should be sustaining you.

You don't have to endure a life that drains you. God's message is clear: There's another way. I thought I was bound by my medical career and hospital job, but when I opened my mind to new possibilities, everything shifted. God was waiting for me to ask for help and make the change. And I found a completely different, fulfilling life.

Your transformation is possible, too, as long as you release limiting beliefs that hold you back. You're in control of your life's direction. God is ready to work in your life, but you have to allow it. Once I shifted my mindset from survival to thrival, everything began to transform.

You can have this transformation. If you're not experiencing it yet, own it, embrace it, and don't settle for anything less. Clearly define what you want in every aspect of your life–physically, mentally, emotionally, financially, and in your relationships. Ask God for what you want, and believe that you can have it.

You're now in Phase 4: The Enlightenment Phase, and I'm proud of your journey. Remember, we all have our ups and downs, moments of enlightenment, and times when we stumble. The key is to keep beginning again.

You got that? Begin again!

Intermittent Fasting: Days 31-37 & 40

- 16:8 Rule: Fast for 16 hours and eat only during an eight-hour window.
- Eat at least three meals a day by following the 2/10/20/30 rule.

Famine: Day 38

- 22:2 Rule
- You will fast for 22 hours and eat only during a two-hour window. This means you will fast from dinner to dinner, or breakfast to breakfast, or lunch to lunch, whichever works best for your life.

Feast: Day 39

- Eat following the feast rule of 2/50/20/30.
- Enjoy a high dose of healthy carbs during your 16:8 eating window. This 2/50/20/30 rule consists of eating at least 150-200g of carbs along with your fats and protein.
- It's important to choose brightly-colored, fibrous foods as your carbs, like sweet potatoes, cabbage, squash, nuts and seeds, quinoa, apples, pears, oranges, grapefruit, grapes, raisins, dates, and figs. Please continue to avoid wheat, oats, corn, rice, and legumes.

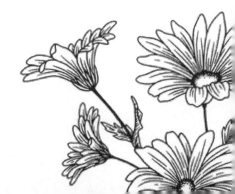

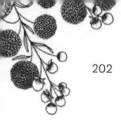

Day 31 Lectio Divina

Prayer of Preparation: "Father, help me to be still and stay still all throughout the day as I meditate on Your Word. Keep me curious and ever growing toward health and enlightenment. Holy Spirit, open my ears to hear God's message for me, open my mind to understand it, and open my heart to receive it."

Ingest: *I will sing to the Lord all my life; I will sing praise to my God as long as I live. May my meditation be pleasing to him, as I rejoice in the Lord. –Psalms 104:33-34*

Digest: Read that again and be curious. See what words or phrases stand out to you, see what catches your attention.

Nourish: Ask God, "What are you trying to tell me?" Then write down what comes to mind.

Grow: Repeat this prayer, "Thank you, Holy Spirit, for reviving my body and reconnecting me to my Father. Stay with me at all times, so I may continue to walk the path toward enlightenment while singing the praises of my God!"

Think about this as many times as you can throughout the day.

Food: Focus on eating three meals a day with the 2/10/20/30 rule within your eight-hour eating window (the 16:8 rule).

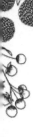

Day 32 Lectio Divina

Prayer of Preparation: "Father, help me to be still and stay still all throughout the day as I meditate on Your Word. Keep me curious and ever growing toward health and enlightenment. Holy Spirit, open my ears to hear God's message for me, open my mind to understand it, and open my heart to receive it."

Ingest: *Jesus looked at them and said, "With man this is impossible, but not with God; all things are possible with God." –Mark 10:27*

Digest: Read that again and be curious. See what words or phrases stand out to you, see what catches your attention.

Nourish: Ask God, "What are you trying to tell me?" Then write down what comes to mind.

Grow: Repeat this prayer, "Thank you, God, for showing me the power of faith. I have changed for the better. I am stronger, wiser, more mindful, healthy, and unstoppable. I want people to see my transformation and be inspired. Please continue to use me, Dear Lord, to spread Your message of hope and possibility."

Think about this as many times as you can throughout the day.

Food: Focus on eating three meals a day with the 2/10/20/30 rule within your eight-hour eating window (the 16:8 rule).

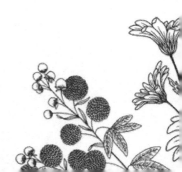

Day 33 Lectio Divina

Prayer of Preparation: "Father, help me to be still and stay still all throughout the day as I meditate on Your Word. Keep me curious and ever growing toward health and enlightenment. Holy Spirit, open my ears to hear God's message for me, open my mind to understand it, and open my heart to receive it."

Ingest: *Honor the Lord with your wealth, with the first fruits of all your crops; then your barns will be filled to overflowing, and your vats will brim over with new wine. –Proverbs 3:9-10*

Digest: Read that again and be curious. See what words or phrases stand out to you, see what catches your attention.

Nourish: Ask God, "What are you trying to tell me?" Then write down what comes to mind.

Grow: Repeat this prayer, "Thank you, God, for Your blessings of abundance. I never go hungry. Thank you for helping me prosper so I may lend and not borrow. The more I can act as Christ's hands to serve, the more blessings You bestow upon me. I am forever grateful."

Think about this as many times as you can throughout the day

Food: Focus on eating three meals a day with the 2/10/20/30 rule within your eight-hour eating window (the 16:8 rule).

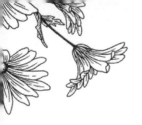

Day 34 Lectio Divina

Prayer of Preparation: "Father, help me to be still and stay still all throughout the day as I meditate on Your Word. Keep me curious and evergrowing toward health and enlightenment. Holy Spirit, open my ears to hear God's message for me, open my mind to understand it, and open my heart to receive it."

Ingest: *No temptation has overtaken you except what is common to mankind. And God is faithful; he will not let you be tempted beyond what you can bear. But when you are tempted, he will also provide a way out so that you can endure it. –1 Corinthians 10:13*

Digest: Read that again and be curious. See what words or phrases stand out to you, see what catches your attention.

Nourish: Ask God, "What are you trying to tell me?" Then write down what comes to mind.

Grow: Repeat this prayer, "Thank you, God, for never giving me more than I can bear. Thank you for giving me choices. Holy Spirit, please stay with me and help me to make the right choices, ones to honor and nourish my body. I love my body; it is strong and beautiful and capable of miraculous things."

Think about this as many times as you can throughout the day.

Food: Focus on eating three meals a day with the 2/10/20/30 rule within your eight-hour eating window (the 16:8 rule).

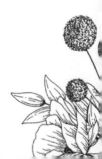

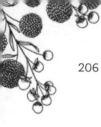

Day 35 Lectio Divina

Prayer of Preparation: "Father, help me to be still and stay still all throughout the day as I meditate on Your Word. Keep me curious and ever growing toward health and enlightenment. Holy Spirit, open my ears to hear God's message for me, open my mind to understand it, and open my heart to receive it."

Ingest: *I have been crucified with Christ and I no longer live, but Christ lives in me. The life I now live in the body, I live by faith in the Son of God, who loved me and gave himself for me. –Galatians 2:20*

Digest: Read that again and be curious. See what words or phrases stand out to you, see what catches your attention.

Nourish: Ask God, "What are you trying to tell me?" Then write down what comes to mind.

Grow: Repeat this prayer, "Wow. Thank you, God, for the gift of Your Son, Jesus. His life gives me new life. I am forever grateful for second chances. The old me is dead. The new me is alive with mindfulness and deep love and appreciation for my body. I love my body so much. Thank you, Father."

Think about this as many times as you can throughout the day.

Food: Focus on eating three meals a day with the 2/10/20/30 rule within your eight-hour eating window (the 16:8 rule).

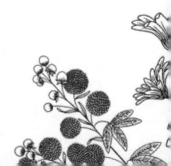

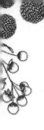

Day 36 Lectio Divina

Prayer of Preparation: "Father, help me to be still and stay still all throughout the day as I meditate on Your Word. Keep me curious and ever growing toward health and enlightenment. Holy Spirit, open my ears to hear God's message for me, open my mind to understand it, and open my heart to receive it."

Ingest: *Forget the former things; do not dwell on the past. See, I am doing a new thing! Now it springs up; do you not perceive it? I am making a way in the wilderness and streams in the wasteland. – Isaiah 43:18-19*

Digest: Read that again and be curious. See what words or phrases stand out to you, see what catches your attention.

Nourish: Ask God, "What are you trying to tell me?" Then write down what comes to mind.

Grow: Repeat this prayer, "Thank you God, for giving me new life, a healthier way of thinking and being. Thank you for showing me how to care for this amazing body You have lent to me. Like Your beautiful child, Maya Angelou once said, 'Now that I know better, I will do better.'"

Think about this as many times as you can throughout the day.

Food: Focus on eating three meals a day with the 2/10/20/30 rule within your eight-hour eating window (the 16:8 rule).

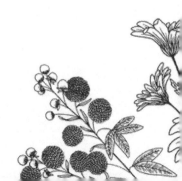

Day 37 Lectio Divina

Prayer of Preparation: "Father, help me to be still and stay still all throughout the day as I meditate on Your Word. Keep me curious and ever growing toward health and enlightenment. Holy Spirit, open my ears to hear God's message for me, open my mind to understand it, and open my heart to receive it."

Ingest: *Surely God is my salvation; I will trust and not be afraid. The Lord, the Lord himself, is my strength and my defense; he has become my salvation." With joy you will draw water from the wells of salvation.* –Isaiah 12:2-3

Digest: Read that again and be curious. See what words or phrases stand out to you, see what catches your attention.

Nourish: Ask God, "What are you trying to tell me?" Then write down what comes to mind.

Grow: Repeat this prayer, "Lord, You have revealed Your power to me. I am a living, walking example of how great You are and how incredible my body is. Please help me to stay courageous and fight against earthly temptations, which only serve to destroy me. I want to be the best version of myself that I know I can be."

Think about this as many times as you can throughout the day.

Food: Focus on eating three meals a day with the 2/10/20/30 rule within your eight-hour eating window (the 16:8 rule).

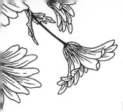

Famine Day: Day 38 Lectio Divina

Prayer of Preparation: "Father, help me to be still and stay still all throughout the day as I meditate on Your Word. Keep me curious and ever growing toward health and enlightenment. Holy Spirit, open my ears to hear God's message for me, open my mind to understand it, and open my heart to receive it."

Ingest: *Let us draw near to God with a sincere heart and with the full assurance that faith brings, having our hearts sprinkled to cleanse us from a guilty conscience and having our bodies washed with pure water. –Hebrews 10:22*

Digest: Read that again and be curious. See what words or phrases stand out to you, see what catches your attention.

Nourish: Ask God, "What are you trying to tell me?" Then write down what comes to mind.

Grow: Repeat this prayer, "Holy Spirit, You speak to me every day. Keep talking. Louder. And show me. I am paying attention now. Lord, thank you. I finally believe in myself because You walk alongside me, go before me, and carry me from behind."

Think about this as many times as you can throughout the day.

Famine Day Food: You will fast for 22 hours and eat only during a two-hour window (the 22:2 rule). This means you will fast from dinner to dinner, or breakfast to breakfast, or lunch to lunch, whichever works best for your life. Make sure when you eat that you are making good choices and using the 2/10/20/30 rule.

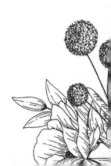

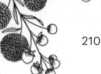

Feast Day: Day 39 Lectio Divina

Prayer of Preparation: "Father, help me to be still and stay still all throughout the day as I meditate on Your Word. Keep me curious and ever growing toward health and enlightenment. Holy Spirit, open my ears to hear God's message for me, open my mind to understand it, and open my heart to receive it."

Ingest: *May the God of hope fill you with all joy and peace as you trust in him, so that you may overflow with hope by the power of the Holy Spirit. –Romans 15:13*

Digest: Read that again and be curious. See what words or phrases stand out to you, see what catches your attention.

Nourish: Ask God, "What are you trying to tell me?" Then write down what comes to mind.

Grow: Repeat this prayer, "Thank you God, I am at peace. You are all I need to be fulfilled, to be content, to heal, and to thrive. Your power amazes me and I am humbled to see how You have transformed me. Please continue to use me as an example of Your miraculous love and power, Dear Lord."

Think about this as many times as you can throughout the day.

Feast Day Food: Enjoy a high dose of healthy carbs during your 16:8 eating window following the 2/50/20/30 rule. This consists of eating at least 150-200g of carbs along with your fats and protein. It's important to choose brightly-colored, fibrous foods as your carbs, like sweet potatoes, cabbage, squash, nuts and seeds, quinoa, apples, pears, oranges, grapefruit, grapes, raisins, dates, and figs. Please continue to avoid wheat, oats, corn, rice, and legumes.

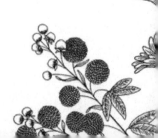

Day 40 Lectio Divina

Prayer of Preparation: "Father, help me to be still and stay still all throughout the day as I meditate on Your Word. Keep me curious and ever growing toward health and enlightenment. Holy Spirit, open my ears to hear God's message for me, open my mind to understand it, and open my heart to receive it."

Ingest: *"For I know the plans I have for you," declares the Lord, "plans to prosper you and not to harm you, plans to give you hope and a future. Then you will call on me and come and pray to me, and I will listen to you. You will seek me and find me when you seek me with all your heart."* –Jeremiah 29:11-13

Digest: Read that again and be curious. See what words or phrases stand out to you, see what catches your attention.

Nourish: Ask God, "What are you trying to tell me?" Then write down what comes to mind.

Grow: Repeat this prayer, "Father, thank you for taking me on this journey of joy. Thank you for the living Holy Spirit, who has guided me. Thank you for the acts and promises of my savior, Jesus Christ. Thank you for Your living, nourishing Word that speaks to me. I now have hope and faith that my body, mind, and spirit are working together to create the desires of my heart. I am beyond excited for my future and I am forever grateful!"

Think about this as many times as you can throughout the day.

Food: Focus on eating three meals a day with the 2/10/20/30 rule within your eight-hour eating window (the 16:8 rule).

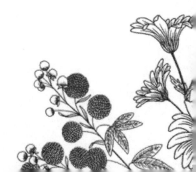

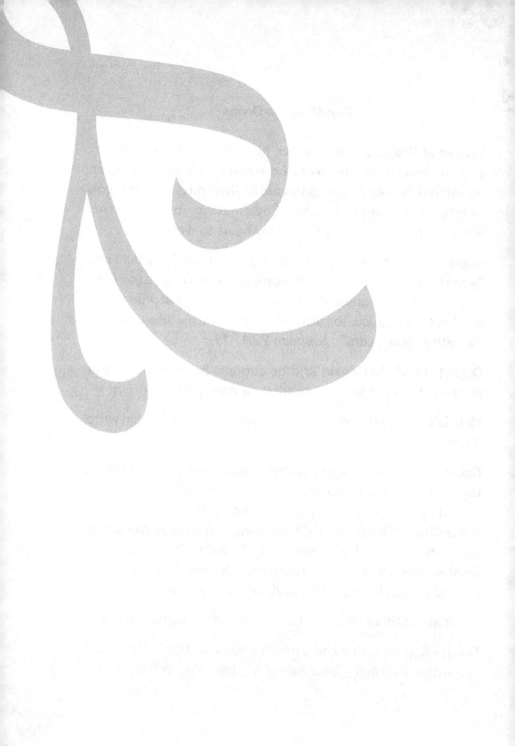

Part 3

Faithful Future

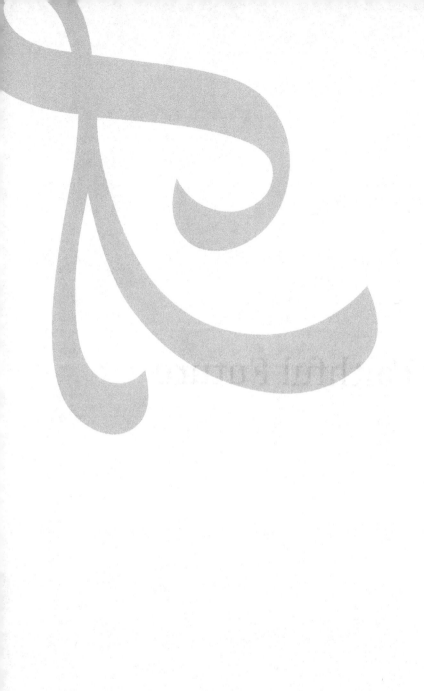

Chapter 15

Thrive in Faith for Years to Come

Congratulations!

You have completed an incredible feat. Please be proud of yourself and don't allow any judgment, guilt, shame, or regret to enter your mind. No matter how messy or imperfect your 40-day journey was, that is how it was meant to be. Find the lessons God wanted you to learn along the way, and figure out what you need to continue doing or change in order to keep growing, transforming, and metamorphosing into your butterfly.

You now see that fasting and faithing are your superpowers for life!

Going forward, make sure when you eat that you are making good choices as I've described in the book and that you are following the 2/10/20/30 rule for each meal as best you can. Don't forget to adjust it to the 2/50/20/30 rule for your feast days.

This is your new foundation for healthy eating. You should fast for 14-16 hours most days. If you are eating enough healthy fats and protein when you do eat, then this should feel comfortable, satisfying, and help you maintain a healthy weight.

If you are physically active every day and trying to build muscle mass and become stronger, then you should focus on eating more protein. Some women need to increase their protein intake to 40-50g per meal. Be mindful that protein can also increase your weight, so figuring out what your body needs will take some experimenting. And remember, your body needs different amounts of macros during different stages, seasons, and phases of your life depending on your activity levels, stress levels, sleep quality, age, and hormone status.

If you have more weight to lose, then I recommend you continue the Enlightenment Phase for as long as you desire, depending on your goals. It works best to do a famine-feast cycle every 10 days along with the 16:8 eating window. Once you are ready to maintain your progress, then stop the famine-feast days.

I encourage you to use the famine-feast cycling for mental clarity when you need to be on your game (like me as I wrote this book), as a gut reset when you are experiencing GI issues, to calm inflammation after "falling off the wagon," when you are traveling and don't have healthy food options, and/or for quick weight loss before important events.

I recommend doing the Freedom Phase (days 21-30) three to four times per year, not only to stimulate autophagy and physical healing, but more importantly, to strengthen your faith and conviction because it requires leaning into God to successfully make it through and reap the rewards.

The key with faithful fasting is to not let your body feel deprived for so long that it thinks you're starving it. This is why I don't recommend chronic low-calorie diets or chronic one-meal-a day-eating. Your body thrives on variation of macros.

Your body will use its resources to "clean house" and thrive if it knows more resources are coming. This is where your faith and mindset come into play. While you are making these shifts in how and when you eat, it's imperative to thank God and lean on Him for your strength.

Here are a few gratitude prayers that I have used during my own 40-Day Awakening journey. You are welcome to use them, and I encourage you to also create your own based on your needs and desires.

1. Lord, I thank you for all the abundance I enjoy on a regular basis. You always give me food to enjoy. I never go without. I have more than enough.

2. Lord, thank you for giving me such an amazing, healthy, self-healing body. Thank you for giving me the opportunity to go without, so I might realize just how blessed my life is by You.

3. I need You, Dear Lord. Every minute of every hour, I need You. Come into my heart and guide me back onto the path where I belong. Lead the way. Give me the power to hear my intuition again; to hear the Holy Spirit speaking to me. I trust You, Lord, that You have given me the tools needed to transform my body back into the strong, lean, healthy, beautiful body You gave me as a child.

Prayers should first give thanks and then ask for what mental or physical attributes you need in order to attain the result you are working toward. For example, I wouldn't beg God to help me lose weight. I would thank God for giving me new resources and the ability to make different choices. I would ask God to strengthen my desire for change and release me from the addiction of sugar. I would ask Him to bring supportive people into my life and thank Him for the ability to influence those around me.

You have influence

Do you realize you are an influencer? You don't have to be on social media making big money to influence people. Your daily actions influence everyone around you. I remember the day I realized this.

It was a brisk spring afternoon and I felt the urge to go running. I live in Michigan and it stays cold until April or May—the weather is very temperamental. You might need a winter jacket in the morning and no jacket by the afternoon. We often joke, "If you don't like the weather, wait an hour."

I looked at the weather app and it said 51 degrees. I thought, Wow, it's really warm outside. I'm totally going. I dressed in capri yoga pants and a tank top. Mind you, I had my winter jacket on a few hours earlier. I started walking out of my cul-de-sac and the clean, fresh air made me feel alive inside. I hadn't felt like that in months because I spent most of the winter indoors or bundled up when I went out. Quick note: I have Raynaud's and Hashimoto's hypothyroidism, so I get cold and lose circulation in my fingers and toes easily.

I turned on my music and started running, or I should say jogging, since I was probably going at a pace of 12 minutes per mile. (I consider it "fast" to run sub-10-minute miles!) Anyway, I was proud of myself for getting out there. While I was jogging, I noticed it was a busy time of day as a lot of cars drove past me. By the time I got back home, I had three text messages from people I hadn't talked to in ages.

"Saw you running, I need to get out there!" one read.

"I can't believe you're out there in a tank top doing your thing. I wish I were like you," said another.

"How are you so disciplined? Teach me your ways!" read the third.

Those texts made me realize that I have influence. The mere act of listening to my body when it told me to go running and not worry about how many months it had been or how uncomfortable I was going to be, changed my future and the future of those around me. When I put my faith in my body that God blessed me with and relied on Him to carry me through, I was able to do something different and move toward a different outcome for my future. The people who saw me doing that also envisioned a different future for themselves.

The key point: To act on those moments! When the Holy Spirit tells you to do something, do it! Don't get stuck in your head and talk yourself out of it. Don't let your mind start listing all the reasons you shouldn't do something or listing all the excuses of why now is not the right time. Those mind games are meant to keep you stuck. Your mind wants to keep you safe, but safe doesn't bring you closer to God and it definitely doesn't bring you closer to health or vitality. Choosing safe, familiar patterns keeps you in your dysfunction, complacency, loneliness, and distant from God.

God expects us to feel the fear and uncertainty and do it anyway. He wants us to trust in Him. When you start living into that trust (called faith) then miracles start to happen in your daily life. Your soul gets fed every time you choose to have faith and believe in yourself. That is what God wants for you. He wants you to be proud of who you are, what you are capable of, and actually live into those promises He made for you.

The last, and maybe most important, component that God wants for all of us is to be a community. God created us to live and play together, which is how we thrive and stay healthy. A study published in the Journal of the American Medical Association (JAMA) in February 2022 concluded that women who suffered from both social isolation and loneliness had a 13-27% increased risk of heart disease as compared with their peers who had community and strong relationships.[40]

According to the surgeon general, "Lacking social connection can increase the risk for premature death as much as smoking up to 15 cigarettes a day."[41]

I see this every day with my patients. They come to me to help solve their medical problems and feel better, but their main complaints are not sleeping well, lack of energy, lack of drive, carrying extra weight, and not feeling like themselves. They often admit to working too much, not spending enough time doing things that bring them joy, putting their needs last to tend to others, not looking to God for strength, and not sharing their struggles with their loved ones. This part is complicated. Many people feel like they are complaining if they say anything to their spouse, or they don't want to burden their friends, or they have lost their connections because of the busy moments in life. In essence, they don't have anyone to rely on, anyone to be their cheerleader, or show them a different life is possible.

Motivational speaker Jim Rohn says that we are the average of the five people we spend the most time with. This relates to the law of averages, which is the theory that the result of any given situation will be the average of all outcomes. In other words, if you are hanging out with toxic, negative people who no longer believe they can have a better life, then you may come to believe that as well.

This is why it was so vital for me to create the FTF Sisterhood, a group of women coming together for the "soul" purpose of lifting each other up and creating a community of believers that

---

[40] Golaszewski NM, LaCroix AZ, Godino JG, et al. Evaluation of Social Isolation, Loneliness, and Cardiovascular Disease Among Older Women in the US. JAMA Netw Open. 2022;5(2):e2146461. doi: 10.1001/jamanetworkopen.2021.46461

[41] Our Epidemic of Loneliness and Isolation: The U.S. Surgeon General's Advisory on the Healing Effects of Social Connection and Community. United States Department of Health and Human Services, 2023.

shows women it is possible to heal and transform. It is possible to live into all the dreams God has placed on your heart. It is possible to have other women support you and cheer you on, and not judge you or want to tear you down.

We have made sure the FTF sisterhood is a safe place—a judgment-free zone of women being their authentic, vulnerable selves being obedient to the calling God has placed on them. God wants us to honor our bodies by tending to them, nourishing them, and believing they can thrive until their last day. This community aspect is a huge reason why the women in the FTF program are successful and have incredible transformations. I invite you to consider joining us online. We welcome every sister of Christ. We want you to experience all God has to offer.

I want to wind down with a few reminders...

Fasting is a powerful tool (it's a superpower!) to strengthen your faith, rely on God, and believe that you are fully equipped to heal and transform into your best self. I hope you have come to realize that this journey of fasting, although not always easy, is worth it.

As you continue to fast, remember that it is a time to draw closer to God, to seek His guidance and presence in your life. Fasting is not just about giving up food, it's also about giving up your own desires and putting your trust in God. It's about humility, repentance, and seeking a deeper relationship with God.

As you fast, remember that it is also a time to focus on your physical health. As I explained, fasting has been shown to have many benefits for the body, including healing the gut, calming down the immune system, increasing weight loss, and reversing insulin resistance. But remember that fasting should be done with the right intentions, and as a means of developing a deeper relationship with God, rather than as a form of self-punishment or self-harm.

As you continue on this journey, believe in yourself and in your ability to heal and transform. Remember that you are fully equipped with the strength, wisdom, and guidance you need to overcome any obstacle that comes your way. Trust in the power of God's love and the power of His grace to guide you through this process.

Finally, remember that you are not alone in this journey. There is a sisterhood of believers who are also fasting and seeking a deeper relationship with God. I invite you to join us and lean on us for support and encouragement, and know that together, we can accomplish anything through the power of God's love and grace.

So, keep going, trust in God, believe in yourself, and know that you are fully equipped to heal and transform into your next best self!

Here is the QR code for my online page of resources, recipes, the online program, and supplements mentioned throughout the book.

Blessings,

Dr. Tabatha

Resources

Here is the QR code for my online page of resources, recipes, the online program, and supplements mentioned throughout the book.

Blessings,
Dr. Tabatha
www.fasttofaith.com/resources

Made in the USA
Middletown, DE
15 January 2024

47891259R00133